RECENT ADVANCES IN ULTRASOUND DIAGNOSIS 5

RECENT ADVANCES IN ULTRASOUND DIAGNOSIS 5

Proceedings of the International Symposium on Recent Advances in Ultrasound Diagnosis, Dubrovnik, Yugoslavia, 29-30 September 1985

organized by the Medical Faculty University of Zagreb

Editors:

ASIM KURJAK
Ultrasonic Institute of Medical Faculty University of Zagreb, Yugoslavia

GEORGE KOSSOFF
Ultrasonic Institute, Sydney, Australia

1986

EXCERPTA MEDICA, AMSTERDAM - NEW YORK - OXFORD

International Congress Series No. 701
ISBN 0 444 80789 6

Published by:
Elsevier Science Publishers B.V. (Biomedical Division)
P.O. Box 211
1000 AE Amsterdam
The Netherlands

Sole distributors for the USA and Canada:
Elsevier Science Publishing Company Inc.
52 Vanderbilt Avenue
New York, NY 10017
USA

Library of Congress Cataloging in Publication Data

International Symposium on Recent Advances in Ultrasound
Diagnosis (1985 : Dubrovnik, Croatia)
Recent advances in ultrasound diagnosis 5.

(International congress series ; no. 701)
Includes index.
1. Diagnosis, Ultrasonic--Congresses. 2. Ultrasonics in obstetrics--Congresses. 3. Blood flow--Measurement--Congresses. I. Kurjak, Asim. II. Kossoff, George. III. Title. IV. Series.
RC78.7.U4I57 1985 616.07'543 86-6235
ISBN 0-444-80789-6 (U.S.)

Printed in The Netherlands

Foreword

The first five meetings 'Recent Advances in Ultrasound Diagnosis' discussed general aspects of the significant advances in diagnostic ultrasound. For the sixth one we have chosen two more specific topics: interventional ultrasound and measurements of human blood flow.

The first ultrasonically guided puncture, using a specially designed transducer, was performed in 1969 at the ultrasonic laboratory in Gentofte, now Herlev Hospital, Copenhagen. Since that first attempt, the new technique has proven invaluable for the wide variety of therapeutic purposes, such as drainage of intraabdominal abscesses, percutaneous nephrostomies, urinary obstetrical applications, etc. There is no doubt that the future will bring an enormous expansion in the number of performers and users of this promising technique. We therefore, have asked a number of experts to review their specific areas of interest and experience. We are especially grateful to H.H. Holm, a pioneer and world top expert for his two excellent chapters.

On the other hand, ultrasonic measurements of human blood flow have brought about significant changes in obstetrics and cardiology, fundamentally because of the tremendous amount of new information quite easily provided by this technique. Gill and his co-workers have been pioneers in blood flow measurements with the pulsed Doppler technique in pregnancy. However, a significant progress is made by the recent introduction of the measurements in the fetal aorta, umbilical vessels, uterine arteries and ovarian vessels. The readers will find several chapters from this field. The new colour Doppler technique is described by C. Kasai, who originally designed the procedure and published the first clinical results.

For both of us it was a real pleasure to work together on these proceedings. However, editorial work would have been very difficult without great help of the secretaries Vesna Balija and Snježana Kvesić.

Asim Kurjak
George Kossoff

Contents

Recent advances in ultrasound diagnosis 5. A. Kurjak, G. Kossoff, eds.

INTERVENTIONAL ULTRASOUND

HANS HENRIK HOLM

Department of Ultrasound, Herlev Hospital, University of Copenhagen, DK-273o Herlev, Denmark.

The last ten years have supplied the medical world with a number of extraordinary imaging techniques such as dynamic ultrasound scanning, CT-scanning and NMR scanning, which on completely different physical basis provide high resolution sectional images with precise morphological information.

However, despite of that and despite attempts of socalled "tissue-characterization" by the above techniques, there will undoubtedly also in the future be a need for a precise percutaneous procedure which virtually without risk can provide minute tissue samples for cytological or histological examination and thereby form the basis for optimal therapy and prognostic evaluation. Furthermore, the percutaneous route represents in an increasing number of cases an important therapeutic alternative in surgery, oncology and obstetrics.

The need for tissue sampling can only to a rather limited extent be fulfilled by gastroscopic, coloscopic and laparoscopic biopsies and explorative laparotomy with biopsy should be avoided if possible.

An imaging technique which can disclose most space occupying lesions and at the same time act as a practical puncture guide would be highly effective and timesaving, especially if the puncture routinely is performed in the same setting as the imaging procedure.

Fluoroscopy in two planes has been found useful but is certainly not especially easy. CT-scanning has also been used to visualize the needle after its insertion.

However, the method can hardly be called rapid or convenient and as stated by Ferruchi and Wittenberg - the procedure takes 1-2 hours.

To use NMR for needle guidance would probably be disastrous.

Dynamic ultrasound scanning on the other hand represents such an ideal method for percutaneous puncture guidance.

The principle in ultrasonically guided puncture is simply that some kind of needle steering device restricts the movement of the needle to the image plane. The scanner is moved and tilted until the target is transsected by the markerline indicating the needle path. When the needle is inserted to the appropriate depth - apparent from the image - the needle will inevitably hit the target. The echo from the needle tip is in most cases directly visible during the insertion.[1,2,3]

A new puncture guide principle is applicable for all dynamic scanners. The image plane is angulated by refraction and thereby the needle can be inserted through a puncture canal directly in the center of the image plane.

Rather few needles are sufficient for all purposes. A lumbar type 1.2 mm needle for all fluidfilled lesions. A o.6 mm needle to obtain cytological material from solid lesions. And one of several types of special fine needles for histological sampling. A fine needle aspiration biopsy is routinely performed when malignancy is suspected in a solid lesion.

After sterilization of the skin and application of local anaesthetic an outer guide needle is inserted just through the abdominal wall to stabilize and allow multiple passes of the fine needle.

The fine needle attached to a lo cc syringe mounted in an aspiration handle is then inserted through the guide needle into the target.

Full suction is then applied and the needle tip is moved up and down five to six times inside the tumor.

The suction is released and the aspiration device withdrawn and handled to the nurse. Procedure is repeated four to five times in different directions.

The material - usually only a small drop - is smeared and stained according to the usual routine.

Based on the usual cytological criteria it is possible with a satisfactory accuracy to differentiate between benign and malignant tissue - but nothing more.

We have used this technique the last 15 years.

The last 2 years we have added a fine needle histological biopsy to our armamentarium. We have used the sure-cut® needle providing microcore biopsies.

The advantages of this technique which has a slightly higher sampling error are that it sometimes can improve the typing of malignant tumors and provide better information about the benign lesions which have caused the suspicious ultrasonic finding. Furthermore, that the tiny histological sections are much faster to screen than the numerous cytological smears. Finally, since usual histological knowledge is sufficient a specialized cytologist is unnecessary.

Based on the fact that complications in more than 5ooo abdominal punctures have been extremely rare we now routinely perform all punctures without any preparations at all. In special cases, however, when a coagulation defect is suspected bleeding time and coagulation time are checked. With large core liver and kidney biopsies the standard precautions are still used.

Only a few restrictions exist regarding puncture routes. Hundred of punctures performed through the gastrointestinal tract and many through the urinary bladder have in our laboratory proved to be quite safe.

Puncture of the pancreas is preferably carried out below the liver edge. However, if the pancreas is not accessible without transhepatic puncture such punctures are performed without hesitation. It is recommended, however, to avoid the very edge of the liver which may be lacerated by the needle during respiratory motion.

Since puncture through the pleura or lung should be avoided a cephalad angulated puncture route is selected for focal lesions in the dome of the liver.

For the same reason upper renal pole lesions are also punctured in a cephalad direction.

The patient should be asked to avoid extensive respiratory movements during the puncture. In some instances - as when the target is very small - it is an advantage to suspend respiration during the puncture.

Finally, it is not wise to puncture aneurisms, but it seems to be safe to puncture pheochromocytomas.

In the following I would like to describe various indications for needle intervention in abdominal diseases and some results obtained in our institution.

A solid focal liver lesion may be a benign hepatic hemangioma or another benign lesion, or it may be a metastasis, f.ex. from a colonic cancer or it may be a primary livercancer.

Occasionally the guided liver biopsy reveals surprising results.

E.g. cytological as well as histological biopsy from an echopoor as well as from an echodense liver pattern in an asymptomatic man showed completely normal findings and a round echopoor area in the liver from a man with a pancreatic cancer revealed slight steatosis.

Even very small focal lesions are detectable by up to date dynamic ultrasound scanning. E.g. biopsy taken from a single 1 cm metastases. The needle tip is clearly visible. An autopsy specimen a week later confirmed the ultrasonic and microscopic findings.

Table I summarizes the results of 247 fine needle aspiration cytology biopsies. The final diagnoses were obtained from surgery, autopsy or compelling clinical evidence.

TABLE I

FINE NEEDLE ASPIRATION FROM SOLID LIVER LESIONS

			Cytology		
			+	-	Insuff.
Final diagnosis	Malignant mass:	222	2o3	17	2
	Benign condition:	25	o	25	o
	Total:	247	2o3	42	2

PV_{pos} = 1oo%

PV_{neg} = 6o%

In a comparative study where each of 77 solid liver lesions had 3 aspiration biopsies as well as 3 sure-cut biopsies performed the sure-cut biopsy gave extra information in 17 cases.

A cystic lesion in the liver may be a simple livercyst or may e.g. be a metastasis with cystic degeneration f.ex. from an ovarian cancer. There are quite a number of other cystic lesions in the liver. For the differentiation of these various possibilities a guided puncture with a 1.2 mm needle is indicated. Puncture through liver tissue is advisable to prevent leakage.

It has previously been considered contraindicated to puncture ecchinococcus cysts. However, recently Sevinc and collaborators from Turkey in 29 cases where they performed fine needle puncture of ecchinococcus cysts had no complications at all. The same result has been found by others.

The puncture technique may also be used as an aid in percutaneous transhepatic cholangiography as introduced by dr. Makuuchi from Japan. With ultrasound dilated intrahepatic bile radicles can be demonstrated and act as a puncture target.

Thereby various irregularities of the biliary tree can be seen after injection of radiopaque contrast medium.

Pancreas, when enlarged locally, is an obvious puncture target.

Since 1974 it has been routine in our institution to perform ultrasonically guided fine needle biopsy of the pancreas to demonstrate possible malignancy. Punctures are performed whenever the scanning shows a solid mass lesion, since it is not possible with sufficient reliability to distinguish between a malignant pancreatic mass and a swelling caused by chronic pancreatitis.

Table II summarizes the result of pancreatic biopsies in 19o cases where ultrasound show a solid mass lesion of the pancreas.

TABLE II

FINE NEEDLE ASPIRATION FROM SOLID PANCREATIC LESIONS

			Cytology		
			+	-	Insuff.
Final diagnosis	Malignant mass:	117	84	27	6
	Benign condition:	73	2	64	7
	Total:	19o	86	91	13

PV_{pos} = 98%

PV_{neg} = 7o%

Simultaneous sure-cut biopsies in 47 patients differentiated almost equally well between benign and malignant lesions but revealed extra information in 15 cases.

When a pancreatic cyst is disclosed a puncture with a 1.2 mm needle is more or less considered an integral part of the study. The puncture is diagnostic as well as therapeutic. Diagnostic since echopoor or echofree lesions may be pseudocysts, abscesses or rarely malignant cysts of the pancreas. Therapeutic since cysts may be treated temporary or definitively through fluid aspiration by single or repeated punctures with possible catheter implacement.

A catheter may be placed directly into the cyst or through the stomach if this is located anteriorly to the cyst. Hancke[4] has treated 19 patients succesfully by percutaneous insertion of a small double pigtail catheter between the stomach and the cyst.

Relief of pain is an important indication for pseudocyst aspiration. In fact, a rather large number of patients are referred to our department for puncture because of pain which usually is releaved immediately.

In a series of 148 patients who had ultrasound performed in our institution during their first attack of acute pancreatitis 19 had developed a pseudocyst of the pancreas. 2 cysts resolved spontaneously, 8 were cured after puncture or catheterdrainage, 1 refused treatment and 8 went to surgery after unsuccesful puncture.

In the last few years it has also proved possible to do ultrasonically guided puncture of the pancreatic duct directly when dilated, pioneered by the Japanese. With subsequent contrast injection and fluoroscopy this technique may give valuable information of the duct morphology and site of stenosis.

Renal mass lesions have been obvious puncture targets since the early days of the ultrasonically guided puncture technique.

However, out of 3ol biopsies in which 83 were from benign lesions, 14 false positive diagnoses occured. These 14 cases, which included chronic pyelonephritis, renal infarctions and adenomas represent far the highest false positive rate experienced in our laboratory. It reflects the wellknown difficulties in renal cytology.

It is therefore of special interest to find out whether a histological fine needle biopsy from renal masses can improve the results. The first series with a o.6 mm sure-cut needle showed too many insufficient biopsies. We have recently for this particular purpose increased the needle size to o.8 mm which seems to improve the results.

A small mass lesion suspicious of an enlarged lymph node adjacent to the aorta as well as a large retroperitoneal tumour represent a clear indication for an ultrasonically guided fine needle biopsy.

From a urological point of view e.g. it is of great importance to be able to detect with certainty dissemination of bladder cancer or prostatic cancer to the retroperitoneal lymph nodes.

A positive fine needle biopsy is a contraindication for a cystectomy and total prostatectomy or seed implantation, respectively.

Table III shows the result of a series of loo fine needle aspiration biopsies from retroperitoneal solid tumours. 1/3 were primary malignant tumours while 2/3 were metastases from a wide variety of organs. No false positives.

TABLE III

FINE NEEDLE ASPIRATION FROM RETROPERITONEAL MASSES

			Cytology		
			+	-	Insuff.
Final diagnosis	Malignant	78	67	6	5
	Benign	22	o	21	1
	Total	loo	67	27	6

PV_{pos} = loo%
PV_{neg} = 78%

Since the ultrasound pattern named a "target lesion" simply indicates thickening of the bowel wall and are non-specific it is not possible with certainty to differentiate between a benign and a malignant lesion. Sometimes this distinction may be difficult clinically, radiologically as well as endoscopically.

By ultrasonically guided fine needle aspiration it is possible to make such a distinction on sonographically demonstrated lesions.

During a 5 years period we have performed ultrasonically guided fine needle biopsy in 78 patients with an ultrasonic finding suggesting gastrointestinal pathology. In approximately half of the cases the lesions was detected primarily by ultrasound. The material gives no information about the number of gastrointestinal masses overlooked by ultrasound in the same period.

In 19 cases the lesion were located in the stomach, in 3 cases in the small intestine and in 56 cases in the colon. The verification was obtained in all cases - the majority by operation and in a small group from the clinical course.

Among the 18 malignant lesions in the stomach verification of the malignant nature of the lesion could not be obtained by gastroscopy including biopsy in 5 patients, although repeated attempts in 2 cases were performed.

Surprisingly 7 of the 4o patients with primary or secondary cancer of the colon were not disclosed by the barium enema.

On the basis of this material we therefore recommend ultrasonically guided fine needle biopsy in cases of incidentally disclosed abnormal bowel pattern. To distinguish between benign and malignant colonic stricture. Also where an equivocal barium study or unsuspected negative endoscopic biopsy is found.

Because of fear of tumor seeding patients with gynecological tumours have previously not been sent to ultrasonically guided fine needle biopsy. However, in our institution this attitude has changed a year ago and solid gynecological tumours are now routinely subjected to fine needle biopsies.

Torben Larsen[5] from our department and co-workers have performed fine needle aspiration biopsy for cytology as well as a 23 gauge sure-cut biopsy from a consecutive series of patients referred to the ultrasound department for evaluation of a suspected gynecological tumour. The two types of specimen were evaluated separately and independantly by two competent pathologists.

The total material includes 13o referred patients. However, in 87 patients the ultrasound examination was either normal or showed no solid lesion.

In the remaining 43 patients the examination revealed tumours with solid parts which could be biopsied transperitoneally without puncturing cystic parts.

26 were performed in local anaesthesia. The remaining 17 tumours were biopsies in general anaesthesia in connection with the

sceduled curettage.

The final diagnoses were obtained by laparotomy in 38 cases which include 18 malignant and 2o benign tumours.

One diagnosis of myeloma was verified by haematological and radiological findings.

Four patients with cytological and histological findings indicating fibromyoma did not undergo operation and have been followed clinically for 8 months, with no evidence of malignancy.

The results of the cytological specimens concerning malignancy were in accordance with the final diagnosis in 16 out of 18 cases. Two were false positives described as suspicion of malignancy and were proved to be a uterine and an ovarian fibroma, respectively. The predictive value of a malignant cytology is thus 89%.

Concerning the benign cytological results 15 were true negatives, one was false negative as the lesion was proven to be a cystadenocarcinoma. The predictive value of a benign cytology is thus 94%.

Finally, 9 biopsies were found to be insufficient. None of the patients had the procedure repeated. The final diagnosis of these patients were malignancy in one case and benign conditions in the remaining 8.

The supplementary histological biopsies in these patients gave a true benign result in 7 cases, 1 was false negative and finally, one was still insufficient.

The correlation between the histological biopsies and the final diagnoses was as follows:

- The 11 positives were true, none were false positives, so the PV of a malignant histologic answer was 1oo% (72-1oo).
- Out of 22 benign answers 19 were true, so the PV of a benign histology was 86% (65-99).
- 3 were false negatives - all cystadenocarcinomas.
- 1o were insufficient of which
- 4 were malignant - these were all detected by the cytological procedure and
- 6 were benign
- 4 of these were diagnosed correctly by the cytology, 1 was false positive and 1 insufficient.

If we add the results of the two types of fine needle biopsies with implicit confidence to a malignant or suspicious answer, whether cytology or histology, we still have 2 false negatives -

the most serious group from a clinical point of view - and 2 false positives. But the total number of insufficient biopsies is reduced significantly.

We feel that the method deserves a prominent position among the preoperative procedures in patients with tumours in the small pelvis.

Another serious challenge for the gynecologist is the follow-up after surgery or irradiation of patients with gynecological tumours. The main problem is to differentiate between post-treatment sequelae and tumour recurrence.

In the posttherapeutic stage the cervical part of the uterus and the rectovaginal area in particular are often difficult to evaluate by pelvic palpation as well as by abdominal ultrasound - which easily disclose tumours of the uterine body and the ovaries.

In this situation transrectal ultrasound scanning represent a useful diagnostic tool which often provides informative trans-sectional images of the pathology in the deep pelvis.

An abnormal ultrasonic finding, however, is non-specific and microscopic verification is mandatory before treatment can be instituted.

In 1981 - together with Gammelgaard - I[6] described a method for precise transperineal biopsy of the prostate guided by transrectal ultrasound.

Torben Larsen and co-workers from Herlev have applied this technique to pelvic masses and used the sure-cut fine needle biopsy system which provides a tissue core for histological evaluation - as well as a conventional fine needle aspiration biopsy for cytological evaluation.

The ultrasound examination is carried out with the patient in the lithotomy position.

After rectal palpation the transrectal scanner is introduced into the rectum - a Brüel and Kjær rotating transducer is used - the balloon covering the transducer is inflated with water. The scanner is started and mounted in a fixture. A sterile needle guiding attachment with several puncture canals is mounted on the rectal tube close to the perineum. A vertical row of dots on the monitor indicates the position of each puncture canal.

The scanner is rotated until the target is transsected by the puncture line. The needle is introduced through the appropriate canal and is seen as a bright echo as it enters the scanning plane. The procedure is performed in local anaesthesia.

The biopsies are performed transperineally avoiding the rectum and vagina. A 21 or 23 gauge sure-cut needle is used and the specimens prosessed for histological investiation using standard procedures.

Furthermore, material for cytological evaluation is aspirated through a 23 gauge fine needle mounted on a lo cc syringe.

The method has been used in lo cases.

1. example

A 52 years old female patient operated in 1978 for an ovarian adenocarcinoma.

In july 1984 the routine pelvic examination gave suspicion of a small tumours behind the rectum. No abnormallity was found by the abdominal ultrasound.

By the transrectal ultrasound examination a solid echopoor lesion 2 x 2 x 2 cm behind the rectum was disclosed.

Fine needle aspiration cytology showed adenocarcinoma and fine needle histology revealed infiltrative adenocarcinoma. Recurrence from the patients ovarian carcinoma (serous type) was thereby confirmed.

2. example

A 4o years old female. Operated July and November 1983 and irradiation therapy was started. The histological diagnosis was squamous cell carcinoma.

In 1984 infiltration in the right side of the top of the vagina was found by pelvic examination. A surgical biopsy transvaginally was therefore performed in May and September showing no malignancy.

Abdominal ultrasound showed no abnormallity. Rectal ultrasound showed a small solid lesion in the left side of the vaginal top.

Aspiration biopsy shows carcinoma of squamous cell type and the fine needle histological specimen shows infiltrating squamous cell carcinoma.

Although our experience with this application is limited it shows that transrectal ultrasound examination allows visualization of the deep pelvic area - where abdominal ultrasound is insufficient - and where palpation may be difficult.

Furthermore, by combining the visualization with a guided biopsy a microscopic diagnosis of the lesion can be obtained. The method seems to be useful in selected cases.

Puncture of fluid collections has been performed for several centuries, carried out with indwelling lead tubes for drainage of ascites fluid.

Nowadays ultrasound has proven most valuable in evaluation of patients with possible fluid collections e.g. intraabdominal abscesses.

A 1.2 mm needle (18 gauge) is used routinely. The diagnostic puncture often provides the physician with important, clinical information.

In a series of 4o4 patients ultrasonically guided aspirations were performed for a diagnostic purpose.

The fluid collections have been distributed everywhere in the abdoman. The size of these collections varies from a few cc's to more than 2ooo cc.

There is no doubt that an abscess should be drained. However, the conventional surgical treatment of intraabdominal abscesses has a few, but important drawbacks. It is stressing to the patients, timeconsuming and it contaminates the hospital environment.

To reduce these drawbacks we have for the past 7 years used the following procedure when a diagnostic puncture has revealed pus from an intraabdominal abscess: An ultrasonically guided puncture is performed. The abscess is emptied completely if possible and the aspirated pus cultivated. The cavity is irrigated with saline several times and antibiotics are installed. A control scanning is performed after 3 days and the procedure repeated if necessary.

Depending on the size and localization of the abscess a polyethylencatheter is introduced guided by ultrasound using the Seldinger technique.

Insertion of catheters through the gastrointestinal tract and urinary bladder are omitted. It should, however, be emphasized that the needle puncture itself is not impeded by the organs mentioned.

It is recommended that the cavity be irrigated with saline the following days, and daily installation of antibiotics continues until the next ultrasound control.

In order to show the position of the catheter and to visualize the morphology of the cavity contrast media may be injected through the catheter.

A series of 1o8 intraabdominal abscesses have been treated according to the principles mentioned. The retroperitoneal group includes pancreatic as well as kidney abscesses and lower quadrants consists mainly of periappendicular abscesses. True pelvis includes Douglas- and gynecological abscesses.

Of these 1o8 abscesses 47 were treated with one or more punctures and 61 drained by means of a catheter. 42 and 5o respectively were cured. A total of 85% were cured.

In 15% healing of the abscess could not be accomplished by ultrasonically guided drainage alone.

After the drainage, approximately 75% of the patients showed a marked fall in the temperature and clinical improvement the following days.

Of possible complications 5 patients had shaking chills a few hours after the puncture and one was treated because of bacteriemia.

E.g. a typical periappendicular abscess containing 3o cc of pus was treated successfully by 2 punctures and antibiotics locally.

In another patient a huge liver abscess was found. The abscess was drained for 8oo cc of pus. A catheter was left in place and the discharged stopped after one week, whereupon it was removed. A control scanning 2 weeks after showed complete healing of the abscess.

We considered ultrasonically guided puncture of intraabdominal abscesses a very important alternative to conventional surgical treatment and it is a routine procedure in our institution.

Ultrasonically guided percutaneous insertion of radioactive Iodine-125 seeds in malignant abdominal lesions and especially pancreatic cancers represents another new interventional ultrasound technique.

A special procedure in which a dynamic scanner mounted in a x-y-z coordinate system is applied.

A maximum of 1o2 seeds were inserted in a pancreatic cancer under direct monitoring using 19 punctures.

Besides ultrasonically the seeds can be visualized radiographically and their irradiation effect demonstrated on a gamma-camera.

We have obtained quite interesting although not dramatic effect in a series of 12 patients treated with this technique.

In 6 cases an obvious tumour-response was obtained and in 2 patients who died 1 and 5 months later of a hepatic abscess and a coronary infarction no tumour tissue was detectable at autopsy.

Ultrasonically guided punctures have been carried out at the Gentofte, and now Herlev Hospital, since 1969.

In more than 5ooo punctures of abdominal lesions including approximately 2ooo fine needle punctures complications have been extremely rare. Among the approximately 3ooo punctures with 1.2 mm needles complications requiring treatment occured in 6 cases. Slight fever e.g. or transient hematuria following the puncture has not been registered as complications.

The two most serious complications was in a patient with obstructive jaundice who required surgery because of bile leak following a gall bladder puncture. The other was a patient with a hepatic aneurism thought to be a pancreatic pseudocyst: After 3 days without symptoms the aneurism ruptured and the patient died. The puncture might have caused the rupture.

Although described in the literature we have experienced no instances of infection, fistula formation, pneumothorax or tumour seeding.

We have only experienced two complications among the approximately 2ooo fine needle biopsies.

Six transhepatic punctures of an enlarged lymph node in the porta hepatis - revealing malignant cells - caused upper abdominal pain. An exploratory laparotomy 6 hours later showed a localized moderate bile leak.

Fine needle biopsies from an enlarged pancreatic head revealing adenocarcinoma resulted in a 1 liter intraabdominal hemorrhage requiring a laparotomy. The bleeding had stopped at the time of operation.

Dr. Ed. Smith, University of Massachusetts, has carried out thorough literature review and sent out a questionaire on biopsy complications to 479 U.S. hospitals of which 45% responded - corresponding to an assumed figure of 63.ooo biopsies.

Based on this survey, Smith found the approximately complication rate for fine needle aspiration biopsy to be as seen here:

Needle tract seeding: 1 per 21.ooo biopsies
Hemorrhage: 1 per 2.3oo biopsies
Infection: 1 per 4.ooo biopsies
Bile leak: 1 per 1.25o biopsies
(This rate is probably inflated by cases of transhepatic cholangiography).
Death: 1 per 16.ooo biopsies
(mainly because of bleeding).

I think it is fair to conclude that the complication rate is very low when compared to the amount of important information gained by the procedure.

I would like to summarize the presentation as follows:

1) Ultrasound is an ideal guide for punctures - not least abdominal,
2) It is a diagnostic as well as a therapeutic tool,
3) The puncture should be considered an integral part of the ultrasound study,
4) There are almost no contraindications,
5) The procedure is virtually without risk,
6) There are numerous actual applications,
7) There are numerous potential applications.

REFERENCES

1. Holm HH, Kristensen JK (1985) (eds) Interventional Ultrasound. Munksgaard, Copenhagen
2. Otto RC, Wellauer J (1985) (eds) Ultraschallgeführte Biopsie. Springer-Verlag, Berlin, Heidelberg, New York, Tokyo.
3. Watanabe H, Makuuch M (1985) (eds) Interventional real-time ultrasound. Igaku-Shoin, Tokyo, New York.
4. Hancke S, Henriksen FW (1985) In: Gill RW, Dadd MJ (eds) Proceedings of the Fourth Meeting of the World Federation for Ultrasound in Medicine and Biology. Pergamon Press, Sydney, Oxford, New York, Toronto, Frankfurt, p 157
5. Larsen T, Torp-Pedersen S, Bostofte E, Sehested M, Rank F (1985) In: Gill RW, Dadd MJ (eds) Proceedings of the Fourth Meeting of the World Federation for Ultrasound in Medicine and Biology. Pergamon Press, Sydney, Oxford, New York, Toronto, Frankfurt, p 321
6. Holm HH, Gammelgaard J (1981) J Urol 125:385

Recent advances in ultrasound diagnosis 5. A. Kurjak, G. Kossoff, eds.

INTERVENTIONAL ULTRASOUND IN OBSTETRICS AND GYNECOLOGY: 8 YEARS' EXPERIENCE

L. BOVICELLI, L.F. ORSINI, N. RIZZO, G. PILU, S. GABRIELLI

Cattedra di Fisiopatologia Prenatale (Dir. Prof. L. Bovicelli)
Istituto di Clinica Ostetrica e Ginecologica II
Università degli Studi di Bologna

INTRODUCTION

Ultrasound has become the method of choice to schedule, perform and guide various percutaneous invasive procedures in obstetrics and gynecology. The safety and accuracy of diagnostic intrauterine techniques as amniocentesis, fetoscopy and chorionic villus sampling (CVS) have been greatly improved and various fetal disorders are now amenable to some kind of treatment under real-time ultrasonic guidance, either for needle aspiration, introduction of shunt, or infusions and transfusions (1,2). Furthermore, pelvic cysts and intrabdominal or intrapelvic fluid collections and abscesses can be aspirated for diagnostic or therapeutic purposes and solid masses biopsied using the fine needle aspiration technique (3). Percutaneous aspiration of human oocytes under local anesthesia has become part of most programs for in vitro fertilization (IVF) (4) while embryo transfer (ET) under ultrasonic guidance has recently been performed (5). Some of these techniques will be described here and the results obtained in our institution will be presented and discussed.

PATIENTS AND METHODS

From 1978 to the end of July 1985 we performed more than 3500 invasive diagnostic and therapeutic procedures under ultrasonic guidance, mainly in obstetrics, but also in gynecology. At the outset, static B-scanning was generally employed but from 1980,when improved real-time equipment was made available, real time scanning became the method of choice. With few exceptions (e.g. CVS) linear-array scanners were preferred in obstetrics and sector scanners in gynecology.

Obstetrical procedures

Ultrasound was used prior to obstetrical procedures for diagnosis of multiple gestation, verification of fetal viability, confirmation of gestational age, detection of fetal malformations or uterine and adnexal masses. The optimal site for needle or trocar insertion was ultrasonically selected on the maternal abdominal wall according to placental location, fetal position and amniotic fluid distribution in order to reach the desired area (pocket of amniotic fluid, cord insertion, fetal parts). The "free hand" technique was generally employed for amniocentesis, after marking the selected site immediately before the tap.

However, a "continuous ultrasound guidance" technique was preferred in difficult cases, placing the transducer inside a plastic bag, and inserting the needle alongside and parallel to it (6). A similar approach was also applied to intrauterine infusions and trocar and cannula insertion during fetoscopy. Fetal therapeutic procedures, as well as placental aspiration umbelical vein needling and transabdominal reduction of multiple pregnancies (7) were always performed under continuous ultrasonic guidance. A real time sector scanner was employed during (CVS)to guide a 16-gauge silver cannula passed transcervically towards the chorion frondosum and to control villi aspiration. A puncture transducer (sector transducer with laterally placed needle guide) was used only for intrauterine prostaglandins administration in cases of marked oligohydramnios and for selective feticide of a twin affected by B-thalassemia. Local anesthesia and general sedation to reduce maternal and fetal movements were employed during fetoscopy or other methods of fetal blood sampling and for in utero fetal treatments. No preparation was generally necessary before amniocentesis, intrauterine infusions of CVS.

Gynaecological procedures

Ultrasound was used for the study of gynecological masses to be punctured and for monitoring follicle growth in patients prepared for IVF-ET. Most punctures were performed transabdominally and through the bladder using a sector transducer with lateral needle guide. In patients with large prevalently abdominal cystic masses or fluid collections, a "continuous ultrasound guidance" technique similar to that described for obstetrical punctures was employed. Transvaginal echo-guided punctures were performed in cases with masses, or fluid collections in the Douglas pouch. These patients in whom the procedure was carried out through the bladder or the vagina were sedated and/or received local anesthesia, while no preparation was generally necessary in the remaining cases.

RESULTS

Amniocentesis

Midtrimester amniocentesis for prenatal diagnosis of congenital abnormalities was performed in 2810 patients between 16 and 22 weeks. The proportion of dry taps, amniotic fluid samples containing blood and abortions after the procedure were gradually reduced with the number of amniocentesis, from 2.4%, 10.4%, and 3.2%, in the first 500, to 0.7%, 1% and 0.2% in the amniocentesis performed last year. This feature is undoubtely due not only to the increasing experience of operators, but also to improvement of the quality of ultrasound examination and the use of more advanced real-time equipment allowing simultaneous monitoring of needle insertion in difficult cases.

Fetoscopy was used for fetal blood sampling in 429 out of 430 cases: B/thalassemia was the indication in 397 patients, a suspicion of fetal rubella or toxoplasmosis in 23, rapid karyotyping in 6, fetal blood grouping in 2 and hydrops fetalis in one. In one case skin biopsy was performed in a fetus at risk for Ichthyosis erythroderma bullous. The overall incidence of spontaneous miscarriage till day 21 after fetoscopy was 3.7% of the completed (10 out of 267) pregnancies, and losses from day 21 to week 28 were 1.5% (4 out of 267). However, 58 patients are still undelivered. In 91% of cases fetoscopy was completed at the first attempt, in 5% at the second and in the remaining 4% of cases it was necessary to repeat the procedure. Pure blood was sampled in 60% of fetoscopies, but the ratc increased from less than 20% during the first year of experience, to more than 80% in the last 7 months.

Placentacentesis was performed at the beginning of our experience; at present we only use umbelical vein needling as an alternative sampling method to fetoscopy: of our 7 cases, 2 were therapeutically aborted, 2 are still in progress and 3 gave birth to healthy children.

Chorionic villus sampling (CVS)

CVS was performed in 40 cases for chromosomal indications and in one for B-thalassemia diagnosis by DNA analysis. Chorionic villi were obtained in all patients, in one twin pregnancy both sacs were successfully sampled. Three pregnancies were interrupted because of fetal chromosomal anomalies and the remaining 38 are still continuing: most of them have passed 28 weeks without complications.

Intra-amniotic prostaglandin administration

Two hundred and forty pregnancies between 14 and 24 weeks were interrupted by intraamniotic administration of prostaglandin F2 and oxytocin infusion, following a diagnosis of congenital disorder or for maternal medical reasons. The abortion success was 100% within 48 hours and 96% within 24 hours. A general reaction to prostaglandins with bradycardia, dyspnea and vomiting was experienced in 5 (2%) of cases.

Reduction of multiple pregnancies

One quadruple after induction of ovulation was reduced to twin pregnancy by transabdominal needle aspiration of the contents of two gestational sacs at 10 weeks. The procedure was uneventful and the pregnancy has now passed 32 weeks.

Selective feticide

Selective feticide of the affected fetus was performed in a twin pregnancy at 19 weeks with discordancy for B-thalassemia by ultrasound guided cardiac puncture, fetal exsanguination and intracardiac injection of 20 ml of air. Continuous fetal heart rate monitoring by real time scanning showed marked bradycardia during exsanguination and cardiac asystole after the injection of the air in the affected fetus, while no significant heart changes were observed in the healthy twin.

The patient was hospitalized for 7 days after the procedure and treated prophylactically with ritodrine. Coagulation studies performed in the hospital and every fortnight after discharge have always been normal. The pregnancy is still progressing and has now reached 28 weeks without complications.

Fetal aspirations

Due to the uncertain results of invasive treatments of fetal fluid collections, we reserved a conservative approach to cases of pleural effusions, ascites or unexplained fetal hydrops. Needle aspirations were thus limited to cases of low obstructive uropathies for diagnostic purposes and to hydrocephalus with additional malformations, in order to facilitate delivery.

Cystocentesis was performed in 3 cases between 20 and 26 weeks with dilatation of bladder, hydroureters, hydronephrosis and severe oligohydramnios, with the aim of evaluating residual renal function in view of a vesico-amniotic shunting. None of the 3 fetuses had a significant increase in bladder volume following urine aspiration indicating that kidneys were not functioning. Therefore all these pregnancies were terminated.

Cephalocentesis was performed in 6 cases of severe hydrocephalus (DBP 10 cm) near term with associated anomalies, in order to prevent cephalopelvic disproportion and avoid the need for a Cesarean section.

Fetal shunting

The aim of fetal shunting is generally speaking to relieve the effects of obstructive dilatations, so that the pregnancy can continue until the fetus is mature enough for delivery.

Vesico-amniotic shunts were inserted in 2 fetuses at 18 and 22 weeks with low obstructive uropathies and slight oligohydramnios in order to relieve back pressure on the kidneys and to permit amniotic fluid formation. In both cases the procedure was successful: the urinary tract was decompressed and amniotic fluid restored, (Fig. 1).

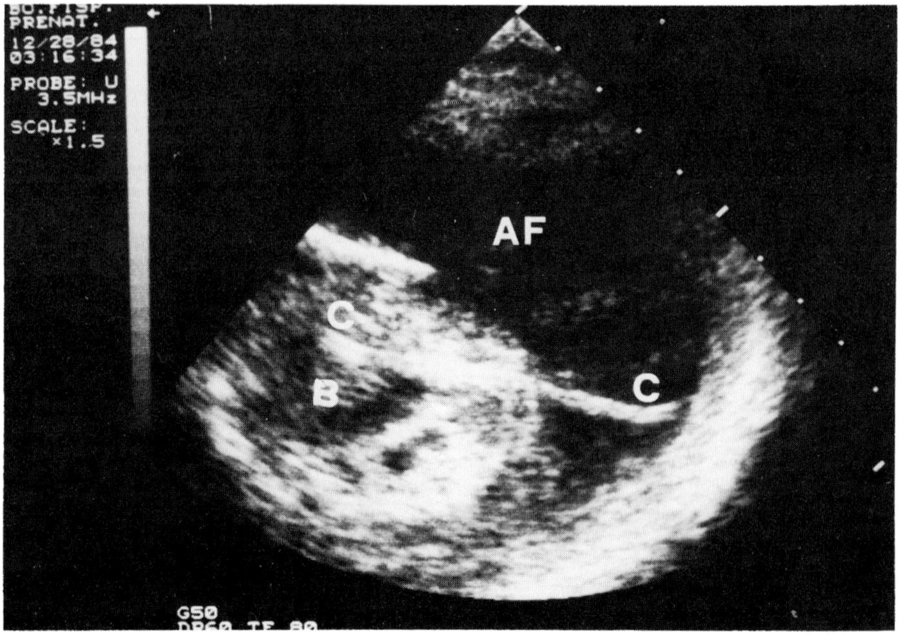

Fig. 1: Real-time ultrasound examination after placement of a vesico-amniotic shunt, demonstrating the catheter (C) extanding from the bladder (B) to the amniotic fluid (AF).

In the first case, the pregnancy continued uneventful after drainage until 30 weeks when the ureters started enlarging markedly, ascites appeared and the amount of amniotic fluid decreased, while the volume of the bladder appeared normal. Therefore we decided to deliver the fetus at 32 weeks after an amniocentesis demonstrated an L/S ratio. At birth the catheter was regularly in place in the fetal bladder, but was obstructed by vernix caseosa. The baby, who showed some signs of prune-belly syndrome had a post-natal uretero-stomy, but died on of respiratory failure on the 4th day. Monolateral renal displasia, bilateral hydroureters with hydronephrosis and pulmonary hypoplasia were revealed at autopsy. In the 22 weeks case the shunting was repeated at 25 and 27 weeks because the catheter had been lost in the amniotic cavity. The fetus was delivered at

32 weeks but died of respiratory failure after a few hours.

Ventriculo-amniotic shunts were performed in 5 hydrocephalic fetuses between the 27th and the 31st week of gestation. We used silastic catheters, that were inserted through (13 gauge needles into the fetal posterior parietal region and left to extend from the ventricle to the amniotic fluid. Their function was confirmed following placement by increased cortical mantle thickness and decreased ventricular to hemisphere ratio, and monitored weekly until delivery. Each case was delivered by Cesarean section after evaluation of fetal pulmonic maturity by L/S ratio. One of the fetuses died because of respiratory complications after the post-natal corrective procedure. One is affected by an intellectual retardation and spastic paraparesis at 3 years at age. The remaining three infants are developing normally at 2 years, 4 months and 2 months of age respectively.

Puncture of gynecological masses and abdomino-pelvic fluid collections

Ovarian cystic masses were punctured and aspirated in 46 patients. In 41 of them in whom clinical and sonographic data were compatible with functional retention cysts a complete aspiration of the cystic fluid was performed for therapeutic purposes.(Fig. 2). In all of these cases cytological analysis was negative and in 21 patients controlled 1 and 3 months after the procedure, the cyst had disappeared. Eight cases were lost to follow-up, while in 12 the cyst reappered, generally within the first month. These 12 patients underwent surgery: 7 had endometrious cysts, 3 serous cysts, 1 a pseudomucinous cyst and the remaining case bordeline malignant cyst.

In one case the cyst developed during the first trimester of pregnancy and enlarged gradually during the second trimester, causing compression. We therefore decided to drain it in order to avoid the need for an operation during pregnancy. More than 800 ml of clear fluid were aspirated and analyzed without evidence of malignant cells. The cyst reappered some days after the procedure but failed to reach the previous size and cause disturbance. The pregnancy is still going on and has now passed 28 weeks.

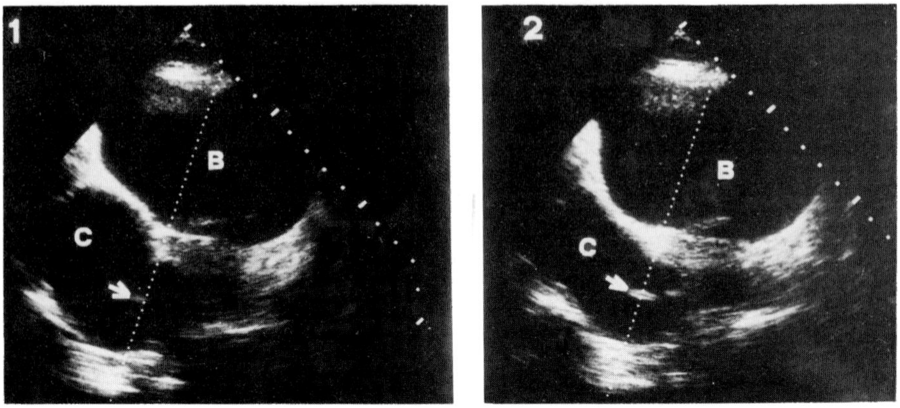

Fig. 2: Transverse ultrasonic pictures showing the operation of a cyst (C) in the right ovary. 1) Needle point (arrow) inside the cyst. 2) Part of cystic fluid has been aspirated. B, bladder.

In four patients the procedure was performed before operation: in 2 with a pathologic diagnosis of serous cysts no malignant cells had been found at cytology; in 1 the cytologic diagnosis was of suspected adenocarcinoma (class IV/V cells), while a simple serous cyst was found; in 1 the cytological diagnosis of adenocarcinoma was confirmed histologically.

Solid pelvic masses were biopsied in 2 patients already treated for ovarian malignancies and recurrences were correctly diagnosed before the "second look" operation.

In 10 cases free abdomino-pelvic fluid collections were aspirated under ultrasonic guidance for diagnostic purposes.

In 3 patients pelvic abscesses were treated by aspiration of the pus, repeated irrigations with saline and antibiotics and subsequent antibiotic therapy guided by the results of bacterial cultivations: 2 of them were cured while 1 was referred for surgery.

Aspiration of human oocytes

Follicular fluid was percutaneusoly aspirated under local anesthesia and general sedation using a 18 gauge needle in 8 patients attending our IVF-ET program. The aspirations were performed 34 to 36 hours following HCG injection (10.000 IU) after follicular maturation had been stimulated by FSH and HMG administration. A total of 15 follicles with diameters between 14 and 28 mm were aspirated. Oocytes were obtained from 6 out of the 8 patients (75%) and from 10 out of the 15 follicles (recovery rate: 66,6%): 5 of the oocytes were fertilized and 3 embryos cleaved and were transferred, but no pregnancy was obtained.

CONCLUSIONS

In conclusion, ultrasound has proved to be the ideal guide for many diagnostic and therapeutic obstetrical and gynecological procedures. However, while the usefulness and accuracy of diagnostic punctures in obstetrics and oocytes aspiration has been proved, present experience albeit promising, is still too limited to allow definite conclusions about the real benefits of intrauterine fetal treatments and the puncture of gynecological masses.

REFERENCES

1. Rodeck CH, Nicolaides KH (1983) Clin Obstet Gynaecol 10:515
2. Johnson ML, Clewell W, Pretorius D, Meier P, Manchester D (1985) In: Sanders R, James AE (eds) The principles and Practice of Ultrasonography in Obstetrics and Gynecology. Appleton-Century-Crofts, Norwalk, Connecticut, pp 289-296
3. Gammelgaard J, Pedersen PH, Henriksen OB (1980) In: Holm HH, Kristensen JK (eds) Ultrasonically guided puncture technique. Munksgaard, Copenhagen, pp 77-81
4. Lenz S, Lauritsen JG (1982) Fertil steril 38:673
5. Strickler RC, Christianson C, Cranz JP, Curato A, Knight AB, Yang V (1985) Fertil Steril 43 : 54
6. Jeanty P, Rodesch F, Romero R, Venus I, Hobbins JC (1983) Am J Obstet Gynecol 146 : 593
7. Mulcahy MT, Roberman B, Reid SE (1984) Lancet 2 : 866

Recent advances in ultrasound diagnosis 5. A. Kurjak, G. Kossoff, eds.

INTERVENTIONAL ULTRASOUND IN DIAGNOSIS AND TREATMENT OF FETAL MALFORMATIONS

ASIM KURJAK, BRANKO RAJHVAJN, DAVOR JURKOVIĆ, ZORAN RELJA, JADRAN JAKOVČIĆ, ŽARKO ALFIREVIĆ, FRANE RUŠINOVIĆ

Ultrasonic Institute University of Zagreb, Pavleka Miškine 64, 41000 Zagreb (Yugoslavia)

INTRODUCTION

Ultrasound detection of fetal malformation is still the most attractive aspect of the use of ultrasound in pregnancy (1-6). It is also essential for both the correct timing and safe execution of a variety of antenatal intrauterine diagnostic and therapeutic procedures (7-11).

Ultrasound scanning has made possible the extension of simple amniocenthesis technique with more complicated intrauterine procedures, such as chorion biopsy, fetal blood sampling and therapeutic procedures in utero.

Some of these techniques will be described here and the results obtained in our institution will be presented and discussed.

MATERIAL AND METHODS

Between January 1980 and May 1985, over 40 000 obstetrical examinations were performed at the Ultrasonic Institute University of Zagreb. During this period, 1487 invasive diagnostic and therapeutic procedures under ultrasonic guidance were performed (Table 1).

Ultrasound was used prior to obstetrical procedures for diagnosis of multiple gestation, verification of fetal viability, confirmation of gestational age and detection of fetal malformations. The optimal site for needle insertion was ultrasonically selected on the maternal abdominal wall according to placental location, fetal position and amniotic fluid distribution, in order to reach the desired area.

All fetal diagnostic and therapeutic procedures were performed under continuous ultrasonic guidance. ALOKA SSD-250 and ALOKA SSD-280 real-time machines mounted with special 3.5 MHz puncture transducers were used (Fig. 1). The transducer was stored in chlorhexidine solution and the skin was painted with iodine. Local anesthesia was never used.

TABLE I

INVASIVE DIAGNOSTIC AND THERAPEUTIC PROCEDURES PERFORMED FROM 1980 TO 1985

Procedure	Number
Amniocenthesis	1266
Chorion biopsy	50
Heart puncture	32
Craniocenthesis	15
Decompression of obstructed urinary tract	10
Urinary shunt catheter placement	1
Ovarian cyst puncture	2
Thoracocenthesis	1
Intraamniotic administration of prostaglandins and hyperthonic saline solution	110
TOTAL	1487

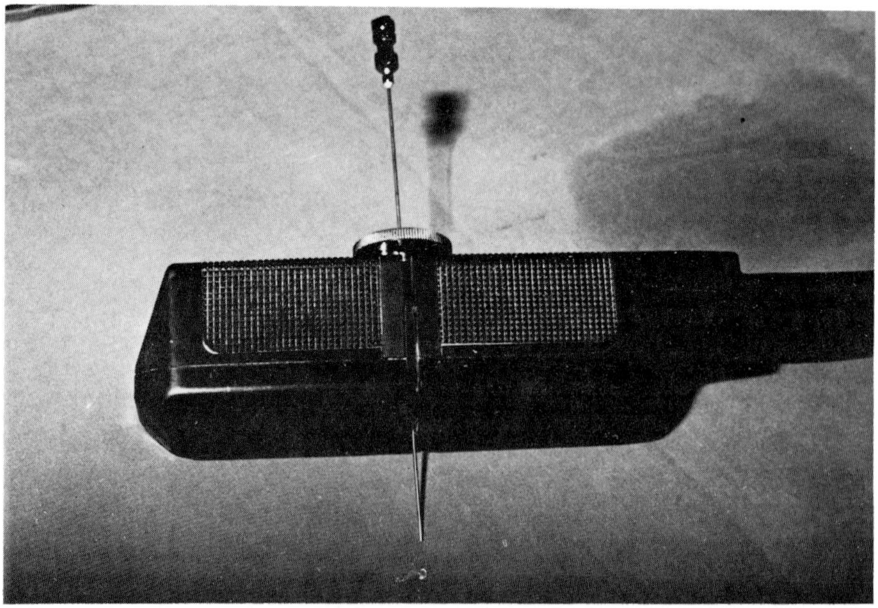

Fig. 1. A 3.5 MHz real-time transducer with needle guide.

An amniocenthesis was performed for sampling of amniotic fluid with purpose of karyotyping the fetus, estimating alfa-fetoprotein, concavalin A, acetylholinesterase and enzyme analysis (25 mm of amniotic fluid is needed for analysis). A 20-gauge stainless steel needle was used for the procedure (Fig. 2).

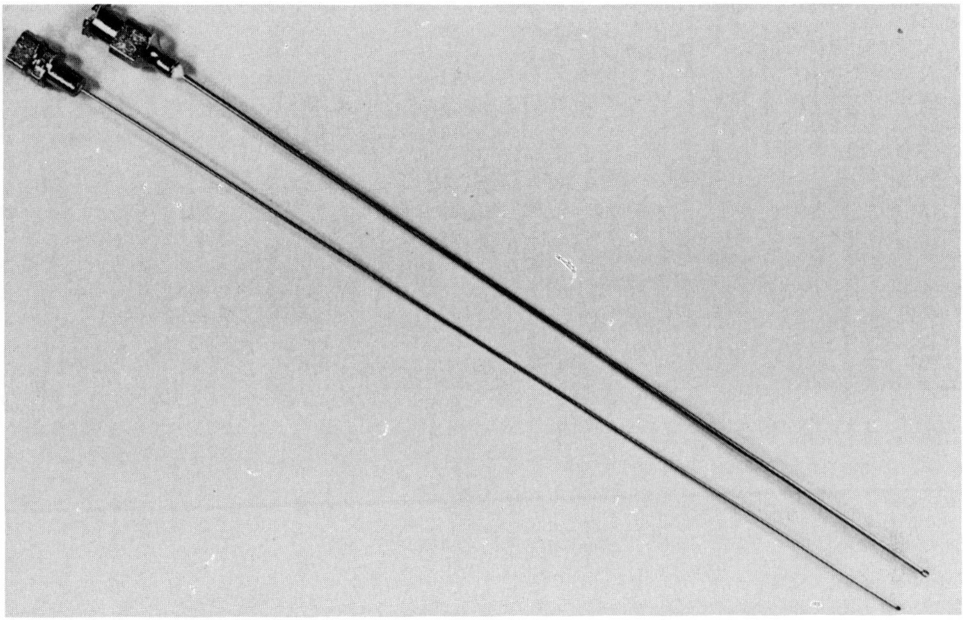

Fig. 2. A 20-gauge needle used for amniotic fluid aspiration.

The tip of the needle could be easily visualized after placing it into the amniotic cavity (Fig. 3).

Chorionic biopsy was performed by direct transcervical aspiration under continuous ultrasound guidance with a syringe and 1.5 mm outer diameter Portex plastic catheter (Fig. 4). In all cases the aspirates were taken from women who were undergoing termination of pregnancy for social reasons. Direct karyotyping were performed in all cases where chorionic tissue was obtained.

Ultrasonically guided fetal blood sampling was performed in 31 patients admitted for termination of pregnancy. A 17-gauge needle was used for the procedure. In each case 10 mg of diazepam was administered to the mother prior to the procedure to reduce spontaneous fetal gross movements. One diagnostic heart puncture was performed at the 23rd week of pregnancy, because there was a strong suspicion of fetal imunodeficiency.

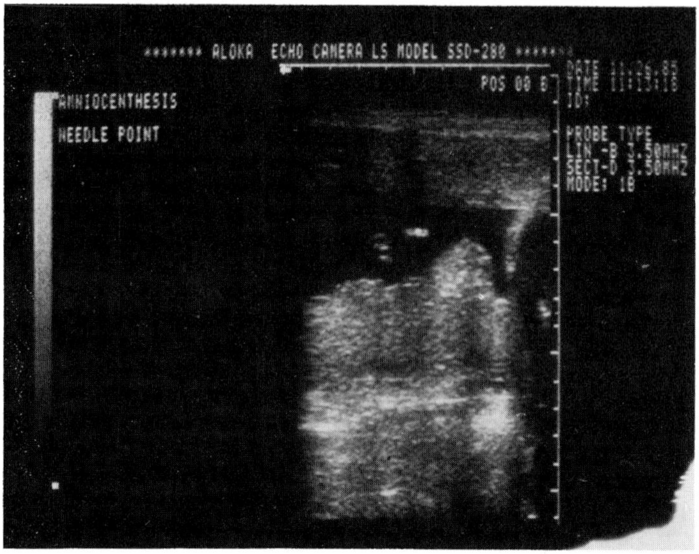

Fig. 3. Strong echo of a needle point is seen in amniotic fluid.

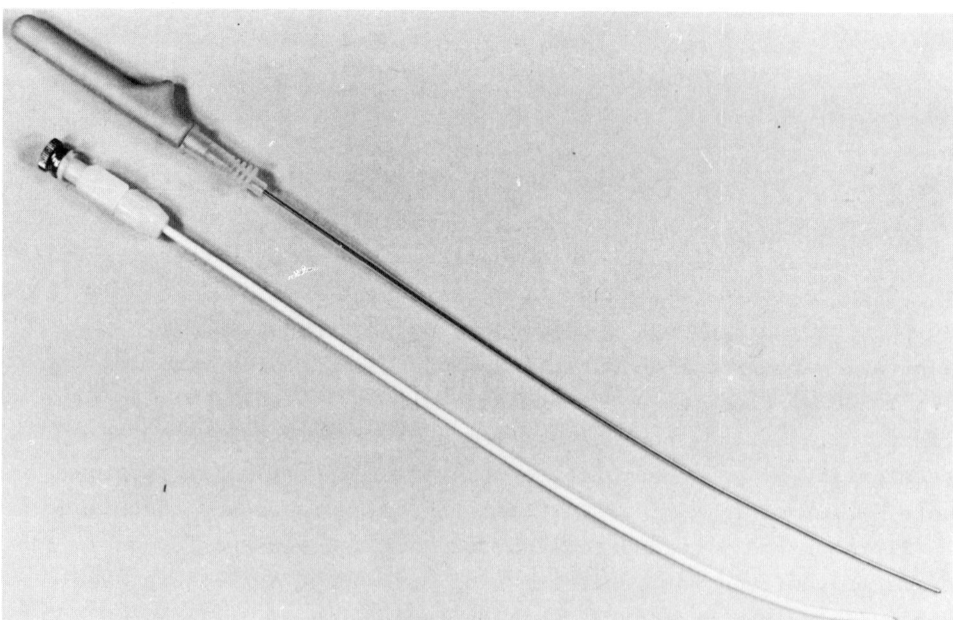

Fig. 4. Plastic catheters used for chorionic villi sampling.

Five out of six skin biopsies performed were carried out before the therapeutic abortion and the 6th one was indicated because of risk for epidermiolysis bullosa. A Tru-Cut needle 15 cm in length was used (Figs. 5 and 6). It can be visualized in the amniotic fluid in open and close position and can be directed to the skin surface of the gluteal region of the fetus.

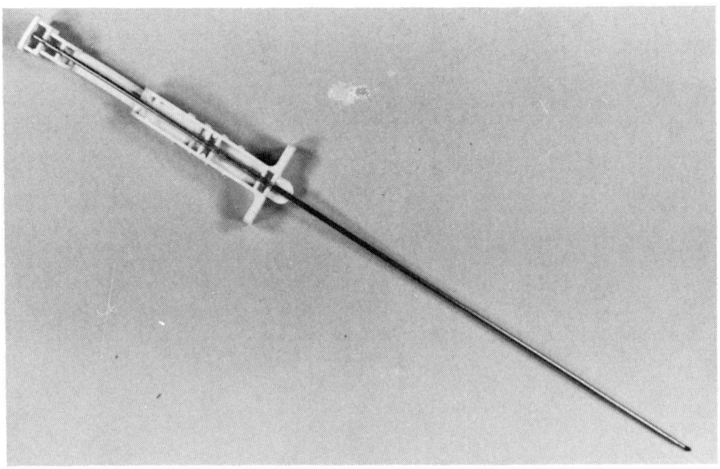

Fig. 5. Tru-Cut needle for skin biopsy. The needle is closed.

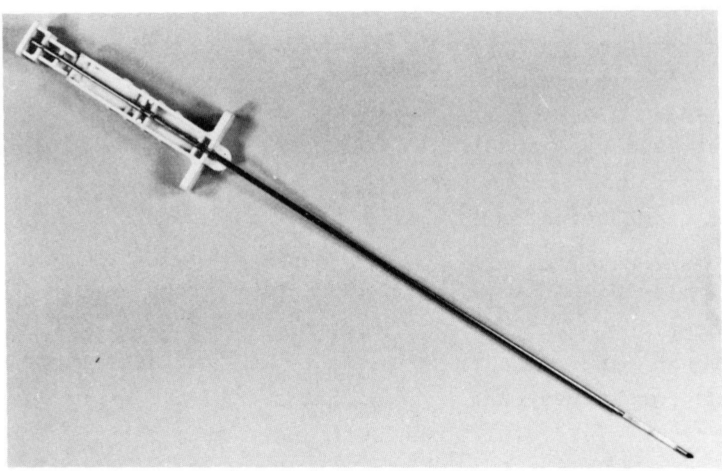

Fig. 6. The needle is opened showing the slit which has to be pressed against the surface of fetal skin at gluteal region.

Fetal therapeutic procedures (paracenthesis, decompression of urinary tract, puncture of ovarian cyst) were performed when indicated according to previously established general and specific criteria for fetal treatment (8, 12).

Craniocethesis was indicated in cases of severe late hydrocephalus when biparietal diameter was 10 cm or more. Decompression of fetal urinary tract was performed when the following selective criteria had been fulfilled: 1) ultrasonically detected oligohydramnios, 2) no other significant abnormality, 3) singleton pregnancy, 4) treatment should commence before 30 weeks, 5) capability of urine production proven by aspiration (after 22 weeks), 6) karyotyping, 7)management should be according to a team opinion and with the patient willing to be treated by a team, 8) management undertaken in high risk obstetric unit with level III neonatal intensive care. Two extremely large ovarian cysts were punctured when largely distended abdomen obviously compressed thoracical cavity.

In cases of fetal malformation incompatible with normal postnatal life, termination of pregnancy was performed by instillation of F_2 alfa prostaglandins or hypertonic saline solution.

RESULTS

From January 1980 to May 1985, 1266 mid-trimester amnocenthesis were performed in 1215 patients between 16 and 24 weeks of gestation. In 18 cases (1.4%), an insufficient amount of amniotic fluid was obtained. In 12 patients, a procedure was repeated with success and 6 women did not want to repeat the procedure.

In 42 cases (3.3%) cell culture failed to grow. In 39 of these patients, amniocethesis was repeated with success and 3 women did not want to repeat the procedure. Indications for ACZ are listed in Table 2.

The outcome of pregnancies is listed in Table 3. 18 (1.7%) patients aborted spontaneously. The percentage of spontaneous abortions was calculated in the group of 1050 women with known outcome of pregnancy.

Chorion biopsy was performed in 50 patients. In 21 cases there were enough tissue for karyotyping. 17 normal female and 4 normal male karyotype were obtained. All women were undergoing termination of pregnancy one to five hours after the procedure. Observed immediate complications are listed on Table 4.

TABLE 2

INDICATIONS FOR MID-TRIMESTER AMNIOCENTHESIS

Indication	Number of ACZ
Mother's age (over 35)	620
Father's age (over 40)	8
Sy Down in previous pregnancies	95
Other chromosomopathies in previous pregnancies	14
Sy Down in family	15
Malformations in previous pregnancies	162
Spontaneous abortions or blighted ovum in previous pregnancies	40
Malformations in family	6
Application of potentially teratogenic drugs ..	23
Exposure to radioactivity	30
Virosis in early pregnancy	12
Parents - quiet translocation carriers	10
Polyhydramnios	51
Oligohydramnios	10
Symetrical IUGR	4
Ultrasonically detected malformation	55
Parents' consanguinity	2
Miscellaneous	109
TOTAL	1266

TABLE 3

OUTCOME OF THE PREGNANCIES AFTER MID-TRIMESTER AMNIOCENTHESIS

Outcome	Number	Percentage
Spontaneous abortion within 3 weeks from ACZ	5	(0.4%)
Spontaneous abortion after 3 weeks from ACZ	13	(1.0%)
Interrupted pregnancy - fetal malformation	43	(3.5%)
Interrupted pregnancy - pathological karyotype	19	(1.6%)
Incomplete records	165	(13.6%)
Normal	970	(79.9%)
TOTAL	1215	100%

TABLE 4

IMMEDIATE COMPLICATIONS AFTER CHORION BIOPSY

	Number	Percentage
Without bleeding	27	(54%)
Slight bleeding	11	(22%)
Moderate bleeding	4	(8%)
Severe bleeding	7	(14%)
Perforation of gestational sac	1	(2%)
TOTAL	50	100%

Direct fetal heart puncture with blood sampling was carried out in 32 cases. In all cases, fetal blood sample was obtained and immediate complication or signs of lesion in thorax or in the cardiac region were not observed. According to our experience the optimal position for fetal heart puncture would be when the baby's back is posterior with the heart close to the anterior wall of the uterus.

One puncture of fetal heart was indicated in woman whose two babies died because of imunodeficiency. The procedure was carried out at the 23rd week of pregnancy and 5 ccm of fetal blood was obtained. All electroforetic and other blood tests were normal. The pregnancy was allowed to continue and a normal term infant was born. The child is now one year old and is developing normally.

Five successful ultrasonically guided skin biopsies before therapeutic abortions were performed. In all five cases, enough tissue for a histologic exam was obtained. One diagnostic skin biopsy was carried out in a woman whose babies died because of epidermolysis bullosa letalis. The procedure was performed at the 25th week of pregnancy. The fetus was found normal. A term male infant was born, who is developing normally through the second year.

In 15 cases of severe late hydrocephalus (BPD $\geq$ 10 cm), craniocenthesis was performed in order to prevent cephalopelvic disproportion and avoid the need for caesarian section (Figs. 7, 8).

In ten babies decompression of obstructed urinary tract was performed by repeated aspiration of urine, percutaneously under sonographic guidance. Eight survived, one had associated limb and facial abnormalities, whereas one infant, otherwise normal, died because of severe respiratory distress (Figs. 9 and 10).

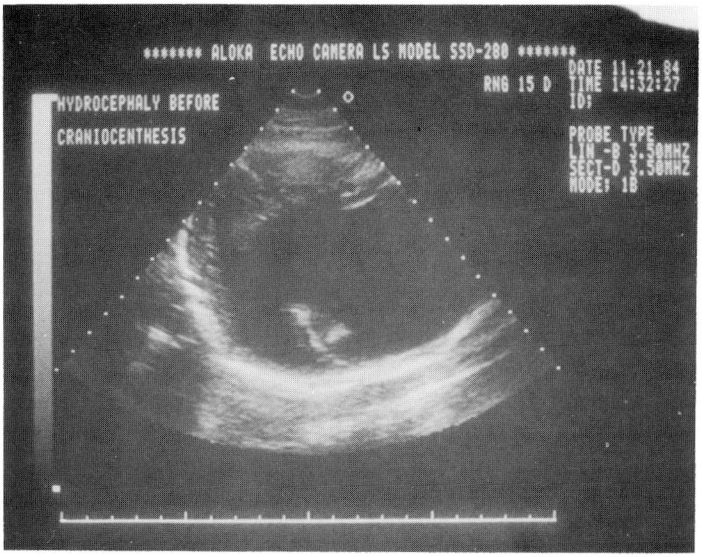

Fig. 7. Severe hydrocephalus detected at 37th week of pregnancy.

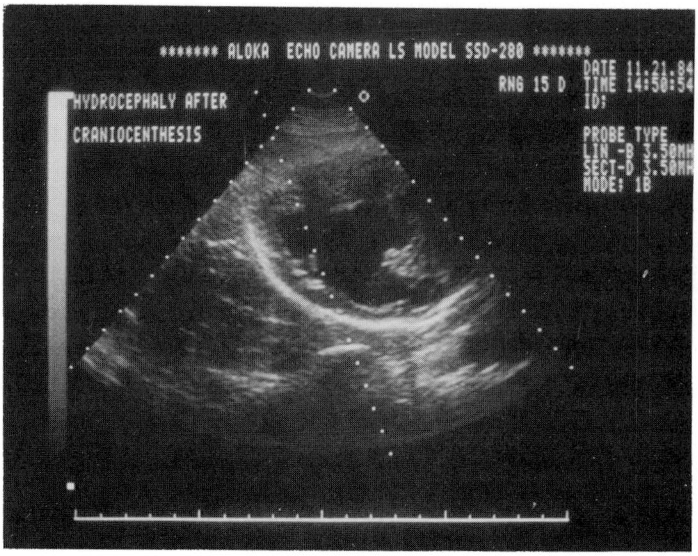

Fig. 8. Cranicenthesis was performed and reduction of fetal head size can be seen.

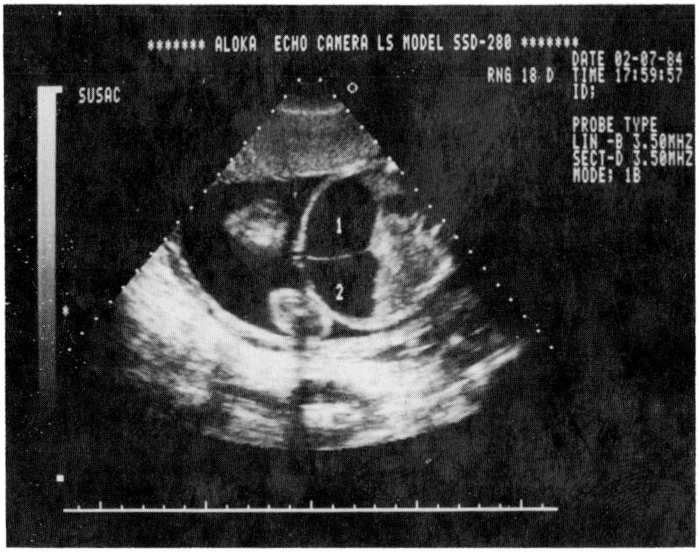

Fig. 9. A case of obstructive uropathy. Two dilatated ureters are seen in the lower abdomen of the fetus at 23rd week of gestation.

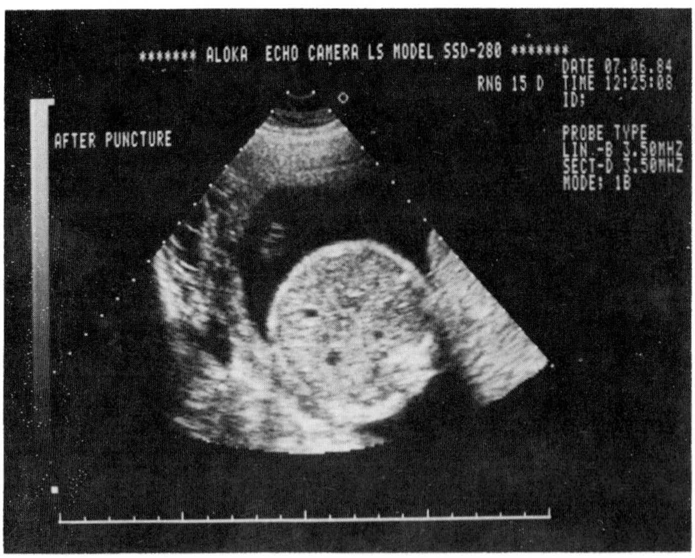

Fig. 10. Aspiration of the urine was performed and transverse section through fetal abdomen shows appearently normal finding.

Sonographically guided percutaneous placement of fetal shunt catheter was undertaken in a 31-week-old fetus with bilateral hydronephrosis due to abnormal pyelo-ureteral junction. Drainage was perfect over a period of three weeks, and at 34 weeks spontaneous labor started. A normal preterm male child was born and a resection-anastomosis of the pyelo-ureteral junction was performed.

Two ultrasonically detected large ovarian cysts were punctured in order to avoid possible antenatal and neonatal complications (Figs. 11 and 12).

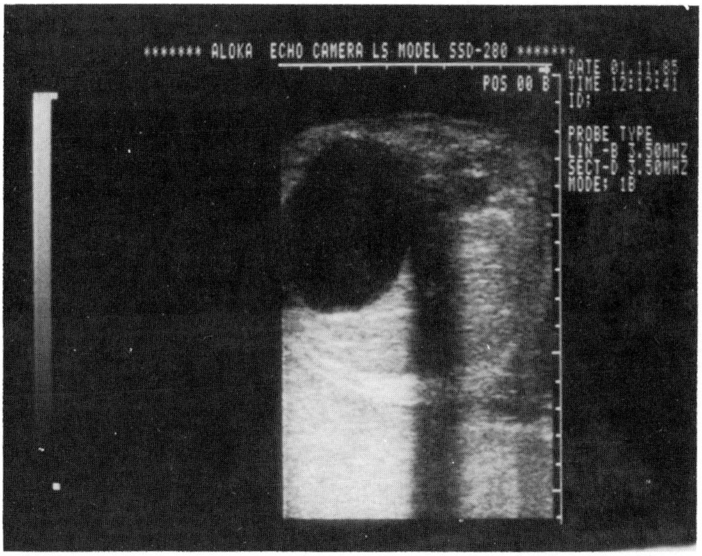

Fig. 11. Large ovarian cyst detected at 32nd week of pregnancy.

We performed the thoracocenthesis when ultrasound revealed bilateral pleural effusions with no sign of other abnormalities in the fetus at the 23rd week of gestation. Immediate cytologic and biochemical examination proved that aspirated fluid was lymphatic. 10 days later, effusion had reaccumulated and the lungs completely collapsed again.

With repeated thoracocenthesis 82 ml of fluid was aspirated. Subsequent examination showed normal development without further accumulation of the fluid. The patient was allowed to go into spontaneous labor. A male infant with Apgar 9 and 10 was born.

At the age of 16 months, he is now developing normally.

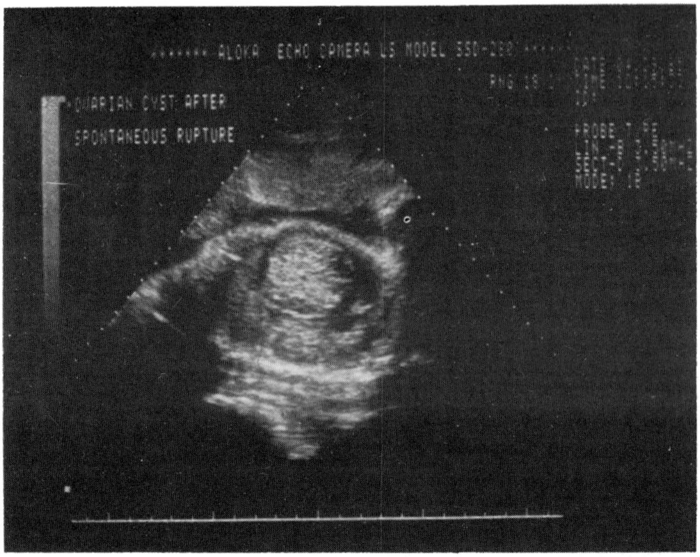

Fig. 12. A 27 weeks old fetus in whom large ovarian cyst was detected. Within few days spontaneous rupture has occured and free fluid in the fetal abdomen can be seen.

110 pregnancies were interrupted by intraamniotic administration of F_2 alfa prostaglandines or hyperthonic saline solution. The abortion success was 100% within 48 hours. No general reactions were observed.

DISCUSSION

Amniocenthesis for prenatal diagnosis of congenital abnormalities is best performed at about the 16th - 18th week of gestation because at this time, the uterus is accessible trans-abdominally, there is a sufficient volume of amniotic fluid and the ratio of viable to non-viable cells appears to be greatest (13). Properly performed amniocethesis is a simple test and the incidence of hazards associated with it is relatively low. The main hazard to the fetus is abortion, but fetal loss and morbidity later in pregnancy may also be a consequence. It appears simple to find out whether amnicenthesis increases the risk of abortion but there are difficulties because patients carry an increased risk,even before amniocenthesis is performed (14). Only few studies have been published which include a comparison group, and are large enough to detect adverse fetal outcome possibility due to mid-trimester amniocenthesis (15, 16, 17).

In previously published papers the frequency of spontaneous abortion varies from 0.9% to 2.8% (10. 15. 16).

The frequency of spontaneous abortion in our group of 1050 women with known outcome of pregnancy was 1.7%. Initially, amniocenthesis was performed without knowledge about position of the intrauterine content. With the advent of ultrasound, the ultrasonographer was allowed to select a pocket of amnitic fluid away from fetal vital parts and the placenta. Although some studies reported that ultrasonography did not reduce the failure rate, incidence of multiple needle insertions, or the proportion of the amniotic fluid samples containing blood (17, 18, 19), some other reports have demonstrated an increased efficiency and safety with this modality (15, 16, 20). In our opinion, ultrasound has an essential place in the safe performance of amniocenthesis.

Amniocenthesis and fetoscopy cannot be performed or give reliable information untill the 16th to 20th week of pregnancy, so there is an obvious need for accurate diagnosis of fetal chromosome abnormalities earlier in pregnancy. Ultrasonically guided chorion biopsy provides fetal tissue samples suitable for culture and genetic analysis at 6-8 weeks of gestation (21, 22). We believe that chorion biopsy will become a powerfool diagnostic tool when used by experienced, skilled experts.

According to our preliminary results, ultrasonically guided fetal blood sampling and skin biopsy are, undoubtedly, very promising new antenatal diagnostic techniques, but its usefulness and accuracy should be carefully eveluated.

Some fetal anomalies require intrauterine "ultrasonically guided" intervention. We have achieved good results in treatment of obstructive uropathies.

With regard to other malformations, a fundamental distinction should be made between unilateral and bilateral uropathies. If one has to manage a unilateral pathology, and has made sure that the other kidney is normal, there should be no indication for intervention either by treatment in utero or by bringing forward the delivery. Weekly ultrasonographic checks will be sufficient.

When prenatal findings suggest bilateral urinary tract

obstruction, intervention may be necessary because unrelieved urinary tract obstruction interferes with fetal development and the severity of damage depends on the degree and duration of obstruction.

Urinary tract surgery should be considered only if the baby is too premature to be delivered, if the baby is unilikely to survive unless surgery is undertaken and there is evidence of decreasing lung function or renal function as well as lung compression.

There are several alternatives for decompressing fetal urinary tract. The fetal bladder or renal pelvis can be aspirated percutaneously under sonographic guidance. Another possibility is early delivery and decompression of the urinary tract ex utero. We believe that the ideal management is early decompression of the urinary tract and continued gestation. Urinary tract surgery should only be considered if the baby is unlikely to survive unless surgery is undertaken and there is evidence of decreasing lung function or renal function as well as lung compression. We would like to stress that the abnormalities of urinary tract are systematically underestimated as a possible cause of morbidity. It was estimated that the average delay between observation of the first symptoms and the dicsovery of the anomaly can be as long as 16 months. Therefore, in 47.4% of patients with congenital uropathies, operation was performed within the first year of life,whereas, only 18.6 of patients were operated within the first month (23).

In our opinion, when the ovarian cysts are ultrasonically detected, it is not necessary to induce early delivery or to perform aspiration in utero except in cases when tumours are large enough to interfere with fetal lung development, and and this occurence is extremely rare. According to our personal experience, we can state that usually no ventilation problems are raised by even very bulky cysts and that the operation, if needed, can be safely performed even a few days after birth.

CONCLUSION

Although ultrasonically guided obstetrical interventions are performed all over the world, it will take years to evaluate their real benefits or disadvantages. It is of great importance to share the information about the usefulness and accuracy of each procedure whether it is already well accepted or whether it is still at the experimental stage.

Today, our knowledge is too limeted to allow definitive conclusions about the role of these procedures in routine obstetrical work. However, its clinical potential should be neither under nor overestimated.

REFERENCES

1. Kurjak A, Kirkinen P, Latin V, Rajhvajn B (1980) Diagnosis and assessment of fetal malformations and abnormalities by ultrasound. J Perinat Med 8:219-235
2. Kurjak A (1980) Fetal abnormalities in early and late pregnancy In: Progress in Medical Ultrasound. Amsterdam, Excerpta Medica, pp 107-127
3. Kurjak A, Kirkinen P, Latin V, Ivankovič D (1981) Ultrasonic assessment of fetal kidney function in normal and complicated pregnancies. Am J Obstet Gynecol, 141:266-270
4. Kurjak A, Latin V (1981) Fetal and placental abnormalities. In: Progress in Medical Ulrasound. Excerpta Medica, Amsterdam, pp 2:77-103
5. Kurjak A, Latin V, D'Addario V (1982) Abnormalities of the fetus, placenta and umbilical cord. In: Progress in Medical Ultrasound. Excerpta Medica, Amsterdam, pp 3:87-122
6. Campbell S, Pearce JM (1983) Ultrasound visualization of congenital malformations. Br Med Bull, 39:322
7. Kurjak A, Gogolja D, Kogler A et al. (1984) Ultrasound diagnosis and perinatal management of surgically correctable fetal malfromations. Ultrasound Med Biol, 10:443
8. Kurjak A, Latin V, Mandruzzato GP et al. (1984) Ultrasound diagnosis and perinatal management of fetal genito-urinary abnormalities
9. Kurjak A, Rajhvajn B, Relja Z, Alfirevič Ž, Žabčič V (1985) Posredovalni ultrazvuk v diagnostiki in pri zdravljenju okvavjenega ploda. Zdrav vestn, 54:299-301
10. Bang J (1985) Ultrasound in needle diagnosis and treatment of fetal diseases. In: A. Kurjak (ed): The Fetus as a Patient, Excerpta Medica, Amsterdam, 277-278
11. Kurjak A, Rajhvajn B, Kogler A, Gogolja D (1985) Ultrasound diagnosis and fetal malformations of surgical interest. In: Kurjak, A (ed)The Fetus as a Patient, Excerpta Medica, Amsterdam, 243-271
12. Harrison MR (1983) Perinatal management of the fetus with a correctable difect. In: Callen PW (ed) Ultrasonography in Obstetrics and Gynecology, Philadelphia, WB Saunders, 177-192
13. Emery AEH (1970) Antenatal diagnosis of genetic disease. Modern Trends in Human Genetics, 1:267
14. Turnball AC, Mackenzie IZ (1983) Second-trimester amniocenthesis and termination of pregnancy. Br Med Bull, 39:315-321

15. Canadian Medical Research Council (1977) Diagnosis of genetic disease by amniocenthesis during the second trimester of pregnancy. A Canadian study. Report No 5 Supply Service, Canada

16. Medical Research Council. Br J Obstet Gynecol (1978), 83 (suppl 2)

17. National Institute of Child Health and Development Amniocenthesis Register. (1978) The safety and accuracy of mid-trimester amniocenthesis. Us Department of Health, Education and Welfare, 78-190

18. Karp LE, Rothwell R, Conrad SH et al. (1977) Ultrasonic placental localisation and blood taps in mid-trimester amniocenthesis for prenatal genetic diagnosis. Obstet Gynecol, 50: 589-593

19. Levine SC, Filly RA, Golbus MS (1978) Ultrasonography for guidance of amniocenthesis in genetic counselling. Clin Gen 14:133-138

20. Kerenyi TD, Walker B (1977) The preventability of "bloody taps" in second trimester amniocenthesis by ultrasound scanning. Obstet Gynecol, 50:61-64

21. Kazy Z, Rozovsky IS, Bakharer VA (1982) Chorion biopsy in early pregnancy: a method of early prenatal diagnosis for inhevited disorders. Prenatal Diagnosis, 2:39-45

22. Ward RHT, Modell B, Petrow M et al. (1983) Method of sampling chorionic villi in first trimester of pregnancy under guidance of real time ultrasound. Br Med J, 286:1542-1544

23. Perrelli L (1983) Prenatal diagnosis of cengenital malformations of surgical interest. In: Calsti A, Astrei A (eds) Prenatal diagnosis and surgical treatment of congenital malformations. Padova, Piccin, pp 163

INTERVENTIONAL ULTRASOUND IN GYNECOLOGY

A. KURJAK, D. JURKOVIĆ, S. BENIĆ, K. STILINOVIĆ and B. FUNDUK

Ultrasonic Institute, University of Zagreb, Department of Obstetrics and Gynecology, "Dr J.Kajfeš" Hospital, Zagreb Yugoslavia

INTRODUCTION

In the past several years ultrasound has become an invaluable clinical method for diagnosis of various gynecological disorders. It can supply clinicians with reliable information about anomalies of the genital organs, pelvic infections or pelvic tumors. However, accumulated experience has given rise to the common attitude that ultrasound can give data about localization, size and origin of pelvic tumors, but is not sufficient for estimation of histological nature of the tumor. Thus, there is still a need for invasive procedures which should be performed in order to obtain samples of tumor tissue for histological, cytological, bacteriological and biochemical analysis.

In comparison with other available imaging modalities such as radiography, CT or NMR, ultrasound has proven to be superior as a puncture guide. Punctures are performed by using small hand-held transducers, and needle point can be visualized continuously during the procedure. In experienced hands, ultrasonically guided punctures are so accurate and simple to perform that some authors strongly advocate that an ultrasonically guided biopsy should be considered as an integral part of the ultrasound examination when additional information about the nature of the tumor is necessary (1).

Interest for interventional ultrasound in gynecology has dramatically increased after Lenz and Lauritsen had described the technique of ultrasonically guided transabdominal aspiration of human oocytes for an in vitro fertilization program (2). This technique is now accepted in most centers as good alternative to laparoscopy for obtaining human oocytes from the ovaries in patients with tubal infertility.

In the following, the technique and experience with ultrasonically guided punctures of ovarian follicles and cystic ovarian tumors are described.

SUBJECTS AND METHODS

Ultrasonically guided follicular punctures were performed in 39 patients, age 25-37 years (Mean 29,6), who were included in an in vitro fertilization program. Tubal factor was the underlying cause of infertility in 37 cases, and idiopathic infertility in 2 cases. All patients received clomiphene 100-150 mg per day beginning on day 3-5 during 5 days and continued with hMG usually 150 IU per day. However, the dose and duration of treatment was mostly dependant on the patients' individual response. Follicular development was followed by ultrasound, BBT chart and observation of cervical mucus changes. The main criteria for hCG administration (5000 IU) was a mean diameter of the dominant follicle of 18 mm or more. The punctures were performed 34-36 hours after hCG administration.

A 3,5 MHz real-time sector scanner with puncture adaptor (Aloka, SSD-280) was used for monitoring of both follicular growth and punctures. (Fig. 1)

After filling the bladder all patients received 10 mg diazepam and 100 mg pethidin i.v. Transducer was placed in sterile plastic bag making sterilization of transducer unnecessary. The skin was cleaned with 70% alcohol. A 17 gauge needle with an outer diameter of 1.2 mm was used for oocyte aspiration. (Fig. 2)

Ultrasonically guided and ultrasonically monitored punctures were performed through full urinary bladder. A needle point was visualized on the screen throughout the procedure. (Fig. 3)

Follicular fluid was aspirated by means of 5 ml syringes. Follicles were flushed with heparinized culture medium until oocyte was found in aspiration fluid. After aspiration of the single follicle a needle point was withdrawn back into the bladder and another follicle was focused in the puncture line on the screen. (Fig. 4) Immediately after finishing the puncture the bladder was emptied by placement of a catheter.

The second group of patients consisted of 25 women, age 20-38 (mean 26,4) years, in whom ultrasonically guided punctures of cystic ovrian tumors were performed. Most of the patients were referred to ultrasound examination because of clinically detected ovarian tumor, and in 7 patients a tumor was found on ultrasound examination without any previous history.

Criteria for patient selection were strictly followed and

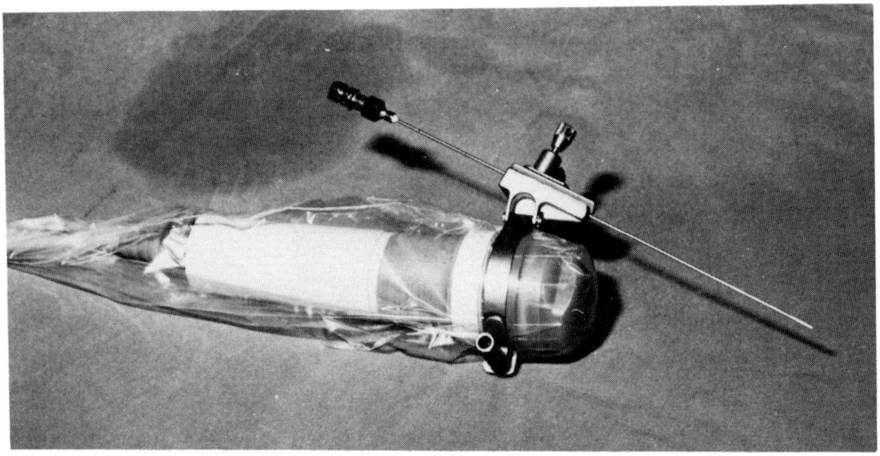

Fig. 1 A 3.5 MHz real-time sector scanner with puncture adaptor. The transducer is placed in sterila plastic bag.

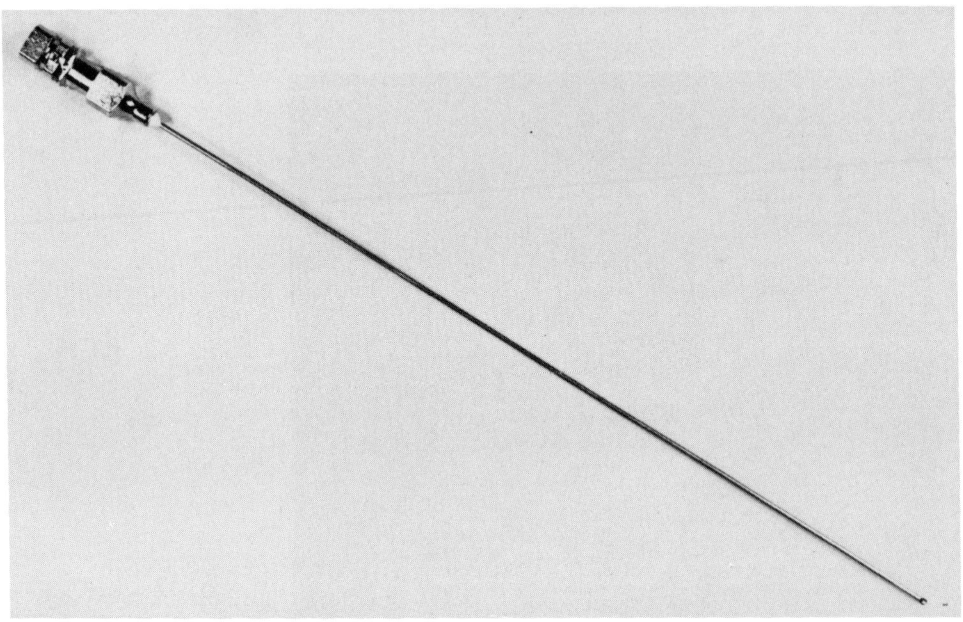

Fig. 2 A 17 gauge needle for follicular aspirations.

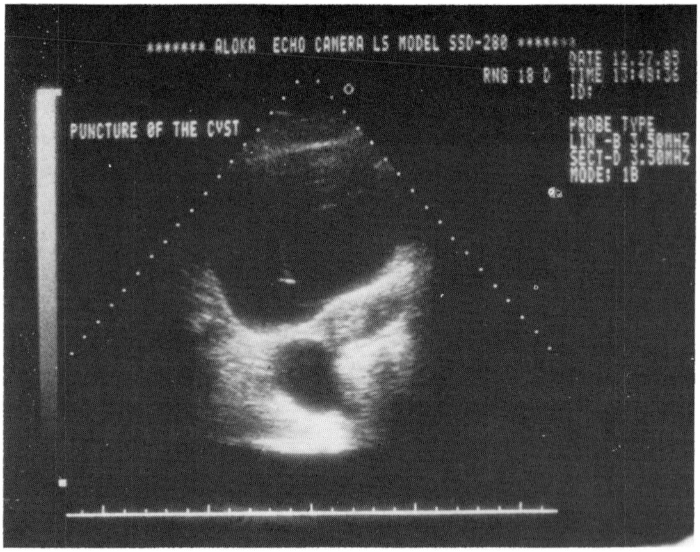

Fig. 3 A needle point in the urinary bladder

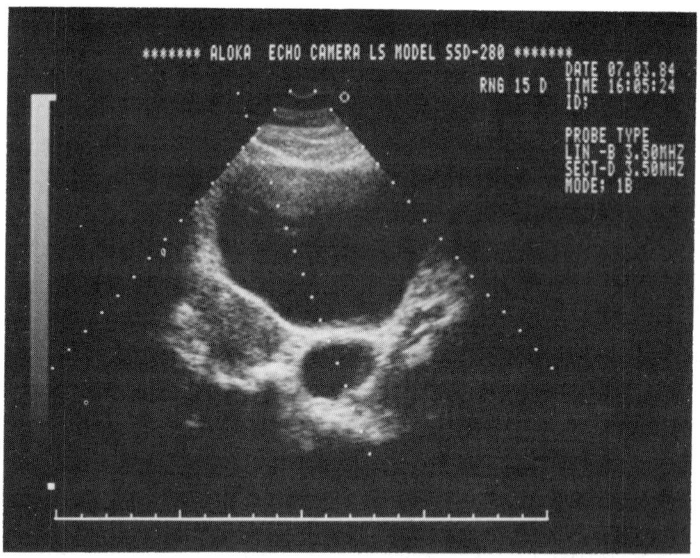

Fig. 4 Mature ovarian follicle focused in the puncture line on the screen.

included morphological characteristics of the cyst, observed by ultrasound, and clinical and laboratory findings. (Table 1)

TABLE 1

CRITERIA FOR PATIENT SELECTION IN THE GROUP OF PATIENTS WITH CYSTIC OVARIAN TUMOR

Ultrasonic criteria	Other criteria
1. unilocular colloid cyst	1. normal blood cells count
2. mean diameter 4 cm or more	2. normal urine
3. thin and clear borders	3. no acute pain present
4. no internal echoes	4. no suspected malignancy

Punctures were performed through full urinary bladder and technique was mostly the same as in case of follicular puncture. A 20 gauge needle with an outerdiameter of 0.9 mm was used for aspiration of cyst content. Aspirated material was sent for cytological and bacteriological analysis. (Fig 5,6,7)

The patients were examined by ultrasound in a week interval after the puncture.

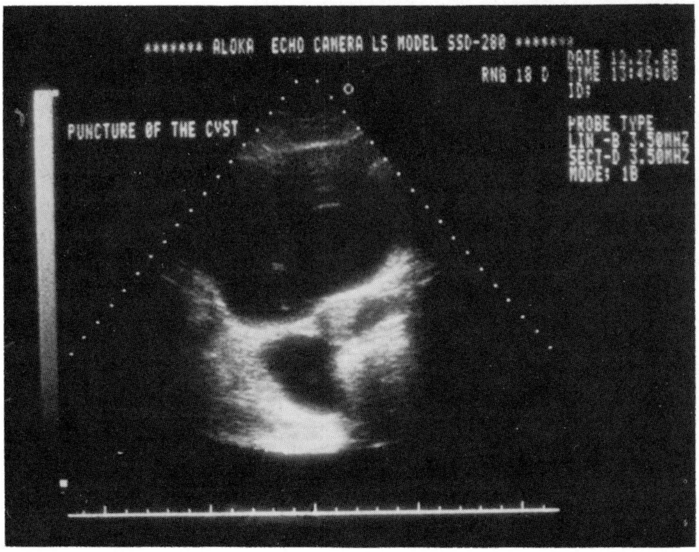

Fig. 5 Simple ovarian cyst before aspiration.

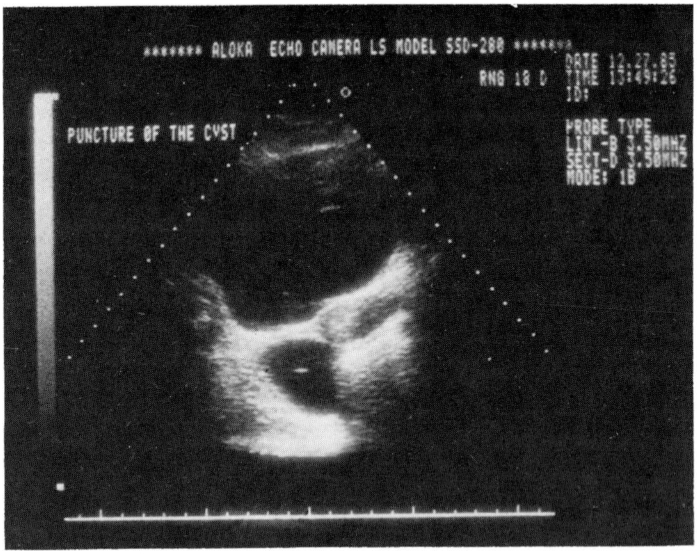

Fig. 6 Aspiration of the cyst. Note needle point within the cyst.

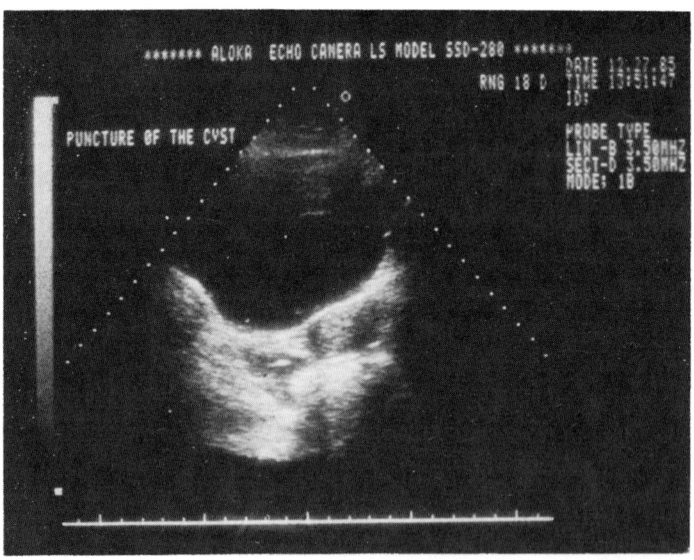

Fig. 7 Complete disapearance of the cyst.

RESULTS

In the first group a total of 121 follicles were aspirated. Follicular diameter was between 15 and 27 mm. Oocytes were obtained from 71 follicle making recovery rate of 58,7%. In one case the procedure was stopped because patient complained of severe pain, and in one case the adhesions covering the ovaries were so thick and strong that pushing the needle through was impossible. In two cases transient haemathuria lasting 2-3 hours was observed. There were no other complications. In the second group all punctures were initially successful and content was aspirated from 25 simple cystic lesions. In 19 cases aspiration was complete, whereas in 6 cases some residual volume remained. Volume of the aspirated fluid ranged from 70 to 220 ml. Clear fluid was found in 17 cases, blood stained in 3 cases, in 4 cases endometriotic cyst was aspirated and in 1 case purulent material was found. Cytological analysis was made in all cases and malignant cells were not found. In one case severe haemathuria occured and patient received 250 ml of blood. From a total of 25 lesions punctured in 15 cases there was no recurrence of the cyst within 1 month after the puncture. In a group of physiological ovarian cyst in 13 cases (65%) there were no recurrence of the cyst. In patients with endometriotic cyst complete recurrence was seen in 50% of cases. 2 patient were sent to surgery because of complete recurrence of the cyst, and in 1 case surgery was performed because of tuboovarian abscess. (Table 2)

TABLE 2

FOLLOW UP OF THE PATIENTS /n=25/

Type of cyst	No recurrence	persistant small cyst	complete recurrence
Simple non endo-metriotic cyst	13	5	2
Endometriotic cyst	2	0	2
Tuboovarian abscessus	0	0	1
Total /n=25/	15	5	5

DISCUSSION

By performing ultrasonically guided follicular puncture, it is possible to organize an in vitro fertilization program as a complete outpatient procedure. This approach significantly reduces costs and is much more acceptable for patients. The technique of ultrasonically guided puncture is simple to perform and is less invasive as compared to laparoscopy. The whole procedure is performed only under slight sedation and analgesia, and there is no need for general anesthesia. Besides, it can be easily repeated if successful fertilization did not occur. Complications are rare and in our group only slight haemathuria was seen in two cases.

The recovery rate of 58,7% is similar to 64% as reported by Lenz (3). Even much higher recovery rates of 87% and 91% have been reported (4,5). The difference in recovery rates can be partly explained by the use of needles wider than 1.2 mm outer diameter (3). Some authors have suggested transvaginal and transurethral approach for follicular puncture especially in cases of deep and low position of the ovaries (4, 6). In our experience the ovaries can be almost regularly reached transabdominally and we did not find strong reasons to change this approach. Ultrasonically monitored punctures have some advantages as compared to the guided one, e.g. there is only one abdominal stab, the entire length of the needle can be visualized in the urinary bladder, an optimal angle to the ovary and follicle can be achieved during the puncture, thus monitored puncture should be preferable.

Although ultrasonically guided follicular puncture is a generally accepted method, there is still some controversy regarding ultrasonically guided fine-needle aspiration biopsy of the ovarian tumors. Despite reliable experience with this method in other areas of the body, there is widespread scepticism to concerning this procedure between gynecologists. The most common arguments against fine-needle biopsy in gynecology are fear of the false negative diagnosis and risk of leakage of tumor cells into the peritoneal cavity (7). Smith has reported results of fine-needle aspiration biopsy collected from 214 hospitals, mostly from the United States. Results from over 63000 puncutres were analysed (8). Only in 3 cases needle tract seeding tumor was recorded and in 16 cases infection complicated the procedure and approximate occurence of these complications was 1:21000 and 1:3333 respectively (8).

It is indicative that only 199 punctures of the ovarian tumors were performed among 63000 puncutres and all were made in cases of metastatic lesions. There were no reported complications in this group, but obviously it is impossible to estimate the potential risk of primary malignant ovarian tumor biopsy on the basis of these data.

Our selection criteria (Table 1) were designed to exclude puncture of neoplastic or inflamatory ovarian lesions. Satisfactory results were obtained and in 19 cases correct diagnosis of simple ovarian cyst was made. In 4 cases endometriotic cysts were punctured which were indistinguishable from simple cysts. In one case purulent material from sterile tuboovarian abscess was aspirated. Ultrasonically simple cyst was observed in this case and all other parameters were in normal range. Used criteria showed that there were no false negative diagnosis of ovarian neoplasm, and none of the patients with neoplastic tumor was punctured.

The purpose of the puncture in our series was twofold: diagnostic and therapeutic. This approach avoids unnecessary surgery in patients who are at low risk of malignancy, and prevents possible complications such as torsion or infection of the cyst. Complete therapeutic effect was achieved in 15 cases (60%) and significant improvement in 20 (80%) (Table 2). The results were better in the physiological cysts group than in the endometriosis group where complete recurrence was seen in 50% of cases.

We are considering the possibility of performing fine-needle aspiration biopsy of complex or completely solid ovarian tumors where risk of primary malignancy is increased. Thinner needles (22-23 gague) should be used in such cases and transvaginal approach should be preferred in order to prevent possible complications of the bladder, e.g. fistula of the bladder (Fig. 8). These preliminary results suggest that ultrasonically guided punctures in gynecology are simple, accurate and safe in properly selected patients. This is a choice method for follicular aspiration and the best technique for biopsy of ovarian tumors. Although complications are extremely rare, its potential for diagnosing primary ovarian malignant neoplasm should be clarified in the future.

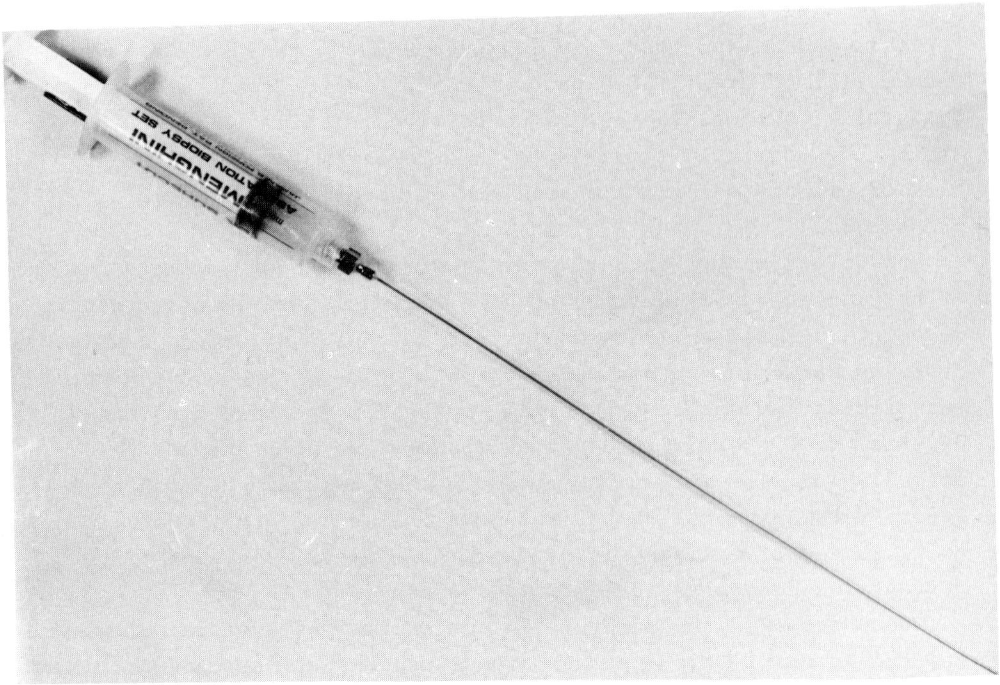

Fig. 8. A-23-gauge Meneghini needle for fine-needle aspiration biopsy of solid lesions.

REFERENCES

1. Holm HH, Kristensen K (1985) Interventional ultrasound. Munksgaard, Copenhagen, p 13
2. Lenz S, Lauritsen JG (1982) Fertil Steril 38:673
3. Lenz S (1984) Ultrasound in Med & Biol 10:625-628
4. Wikland M, Hamberger L (1984) Le Journal Francais d'Echographie 2:83
5. Feichtinger W (1984) In: Kurjak A, Kossoff G (eds) Recent advances in ultrasound diagnosis. Excerpta Medica, Amsterdam p 218
6. Parsons J (1985) Personal comunication
7. Jensen F (1985) In: Holm HH, Kristensen K (eds) Interventional ultrasound. Munksgaard, Copenhagen, p 114
8. Smith EH (1984) Ultrasound Med & Biol 10:629-634.

Recent advances in ultrasound diagnosis 5. A. Kurjak, G. Kossoff, eds.

PROGRESS IN INTERVENTIONAL ECHOCARDIOGRAPHY

I. ČIKEŠ, B. BREYER, B. FEREK-PETRIĆ
Institute of Cardiovascular Disease, University Hospital Rebro, Zagreb, Yugoslavia

INTRODUCTION

Interventional echocardiography can be defined as the use of echocardiography for guiding or assessing various interventions in cardiology, making them safer and less invasive.

Several interventional methods in cardiology can be guided by echocardiography: pericardiocentesis, percutaneous pericardial biopsy, percutaneous pericardial fenestration, endomyocardial biopsy, cardiac catheterization, introduction of pacemaker electrodes and electrodes for electrophysiological studies, intracardiac echocardiography, transesophageal echocardiography, transseptal left atrial catheterization, balloon septosomy, intraoperative echocardiography and laser phototherapy.

Interventions which can be assessed by echocardiography are: percutaneous transluminal coronary angioplasty, streptokinase thrombolysis, contrast studies, myocardial perfusion studies, drug studies, exercise echocardiography and intraoperative echocardiography.

Over the last few years our laboratory has been involved in developing intrapericardial interventions directed by ultrasound. Recently, a new method of cardiac catheterization and the introduction of pacemaker electrodes and electrodes for electrophysiological studies under echocardiographic guidance have been developed.

PERICARDIOCENTESIS GUIDED BY ECHOCARDIOGRAPHY

Although introduced in 1840, pericardiocentesis is still a procedure with a high risk of morbidity and mortality. Before the era of echocardiography, complications were frequently reported. The introduction of echocardiography in the routine diagnosis of pericardial effusion is a most important advance in reducing the hazards of pericardiocentesis. Since echocardiography can provide a reliable diagnosis and determine the approximate amount, distribution and possible loculation of pericardial fluid, it is essential in the selection of patients for pericardiocentesis. And on this basis the optimal puncture site can be determined.

Several methods have been reported which claim to reduce the potential risks of pericardiocentesis (Fig. 1) (Cikes & Ernst).

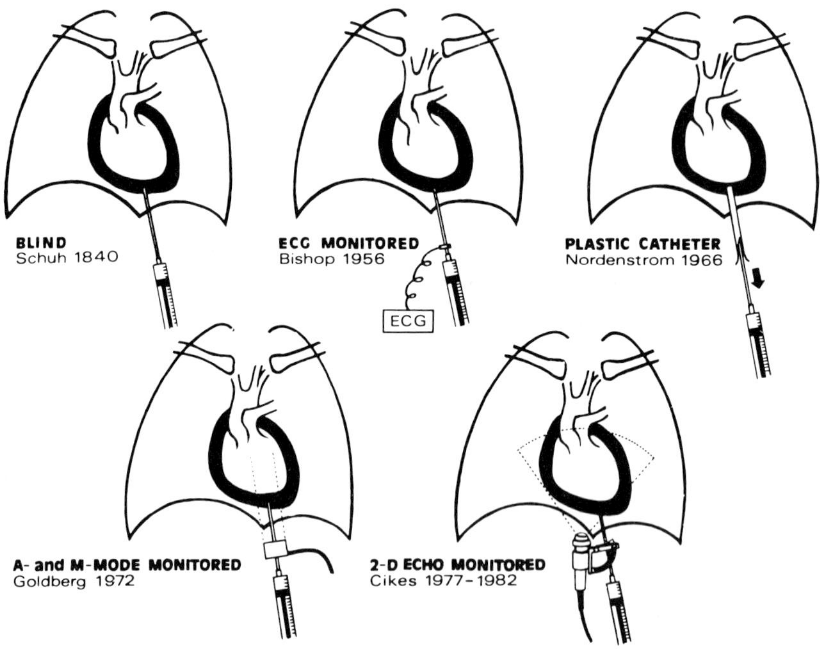

Fig. 1 Different techniques of pericardiocentesis

Fluoroscopic guidance of the puncture needle is not a reliable method because it cannot differentiate pericardial effusion from the cardiac mass. Electrocardiographic monitoring of pericardiocentesis described by Bishop and coworkers may give a spurious feeling of safety and usually registers already existing injury. Plastic catheters introduced into the pericardial sac over or through the needle or guide wire is much safer. In 1972, Goldberg & Pollock used a special transducer with a hole in the center to direct the needle during pericardiocentesis under A- and M- mode display as an echo arising at the needle tip-fluid interface. In 1 out of 6 reported patients ventricular puncture was performed. As is seen from the literature, this method was of no further interest in cardiology. The main disadvantage of pericardiocentesis guided under A- and M- mode control is the lack of spatial orientation.

In order to ensure safe diagnostic and therapeutic pericardiocentesis we have, over the last 5 years, guided the needle for pericardiocentesis by 2-dimensional echocardiography in 30 patients with pericardial effusion. All the patients had moderate to large pericardial effusions. For safe pericardiocentesis it is essential to position the needle in the scanning plane. If part of the needle is outside the scanning plane the location of the needle tip is misinterpreted (Fig. 2). The position of the needle tip can be

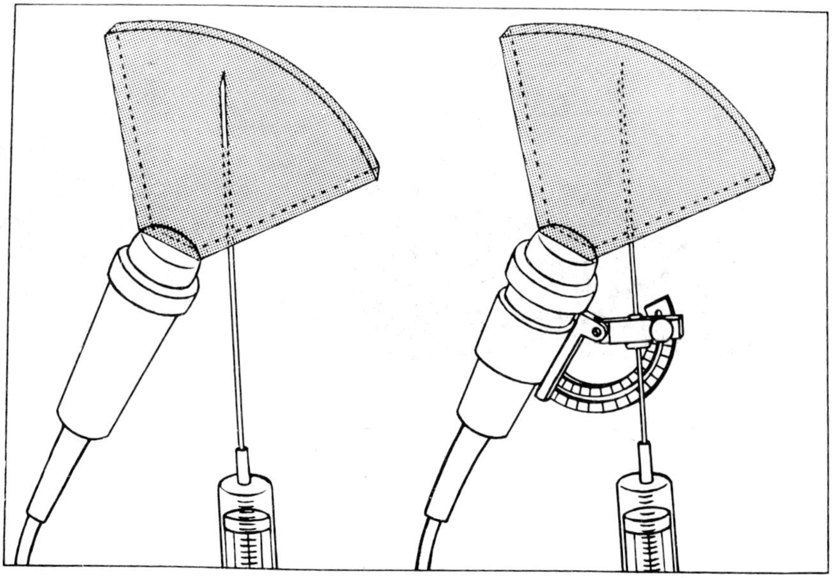

Fig. 2 Identification of needle tip
The point where the needle leaves the scanning plane may be misinterpreted as the needle tip. A puncture adaptor (right) mounted on the transducer ensures that the needle is kept in the scanning plane at an adjustable angle to the transducer.

confirmed by a contrast study - instillation of 2 to 5 ml of sterile saline or pericardial fluid through the needle. If a contrast jet appears at the location of the presumed needle tip, it can be considered the true tip. Besides the classical subxyphoid approach we perform pericardiocentesis through the posterior or lateral thoracic wall in patients with concomitant pleural effusion (Fig. 3). We find this approach to be most convenient provided a

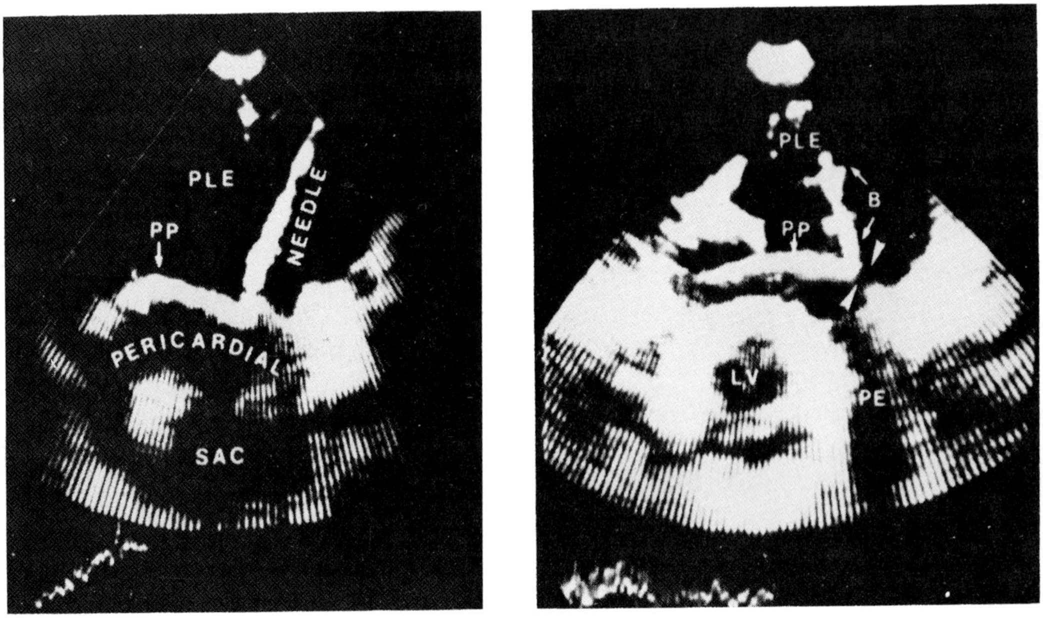

Fig. 3 Pericardial window
A: The needle for pericardiocentesis in pleural effusion (PLE) reaching perietal pericardium (PP). B. Bioptom (B) and window (arrows) in the parietal pericardium created during pericardial biopsy. PE: pericardial effusion LV, left ventricle.

large pleural effusion assures a large echo-free corridor to the parietal pericardium. In addition, the largest amount of pericardial fluid usually collects behind the left posterior ventricular wall and the cardiac apex moves away from the needle in systole, reducing the risk of cardiac damage. After entering the pericardial sac the needle should be replaced by a plastic catheter.

The position of the needle or replacement catheter should be monitored continuously during the procedure and the needle repositioned if necessary. In 1 out of our 30 patients a ventricular puncture with intrapericardial bleeding occured, requiring immediate thoracotomy. In this patient an apical approach was used because an enlarged nodular liver thwarted the subxyphoid approach.

Recently, we have constructed a puncture adaptor mounted on the phased array transducer (see Fig. 2). The adaptor ensures that the needle follows the predetermined needle path and stays in the scanning plane. This eliminates the possibility of misinterpretation of the position of the needle tip. The angle of the needle path can be adjusted. Particular attention should be paid to preparation of the patient, adequate sterilization of instruments and electrical safety precautions. We believe that the technique described can eliminate the risk of cardiac damage during pericardiocentesis.

PERCUTANEOUS PERICARDIAL BIOPSY AND FENESTRATION

Diagnostic pericardiocentesis enables etiologic diagnosis in less than one third of patients with pericardial effusion. Thus, in many cases thoracotomy with pericardial biopsy remains the definitive diagnostic solution.

In an attempt to avoid thoracotomy and general anesthesia for histologic diagnosis of pericardial lesions in patients with pericardial effusion we have introduced a new technique of percutaneous pericardial biopsy and pericardial fenestration under 2-dimensional echocardiographic guidance. The same technique as described for pericardiocentesis was used. Pericardial biopsy was performed in 6 patients, while a pericardial window was created in 2 patients. In patients with concomitant left pleural effusion, the posterior or lateral thoracic approach was preffered, as in pericardiocentesis (Fig. 3). A disposable Trucut Travenel needle with a 15.2 cm cannula length and 20 mm specimen notch was used. After the pericardial specimen was taken the hole was enlarged to a pericardial window and pericardial fluid drained into the pleural space. A pericardial window created during biopsy for decompression can save repeated pericardiocentesis in recurrent pericardial effusion with tamponade. In all patients an adequate tissue specimen for histological analysis was obtained and proper histological diagnosis was made. It is believed that the adaptor described will refine the biopsy technique and improve its safety.

CARDIAC CATHETERIZATION GUIDED BY ULTRASOUND

To avoid the well-known disadvantages of conventional X-ray guided cardiac catherization, we have developed a system for ultrasonic guidance of the catheters in cardiac cavities. The main disadvantages of X-ray guided cardiac catheterization are: X-ray irradiation of the patient and laboratory staff, injection of a large volume of iodine contrast with its toxic and hemodynamic effects, lack of spatial orientation, lack of detailed anatomical data, the high cost of equipment, space and installation. This method can therefore be used only in a limited number of cardiac centers.

Ultrasonically guided cardiac catheterization can overcome all these disadvantages. The introduction of catheters into cardiac cavities is not, in itself, the most invasive part of cardiac catheterization, as arrhythmias can now be kept well under control. Two-dimensional echocardiography provides superior morphologic information of the heart in real-time which could not be obtained by other techniques. However, in some patients we need additional data on intracardiac pressures and oxymetric data for the calculation of intracardiac shunts in order to make a definitive cardiac diagnosis and clinical decisions.

The portions of the catheter which are in the scanning plane can be ultrasonically imaged in the cardiac cavities due to their different acoustic impedance. In order to obtain intracardiac pressure measurements and blood samples for a precise position it is essential to identify the catheter tip. There are several possible sources of misinterpretation of the catheter tip. Each point at which the catheter enters or leaves the scanning plane can be misinterpreted as the tip. Some cardiac structures such as the papillary muscles, trabeculae, chordae tendineae and the valvular apparatus can also be sources of misinterpretation of the catheter tip. A possible problem may also be phantom or spurious echoes.

We have tested several methods for the identification of the catheter tip. Injection of contrast through the catheter has proved to be an unreliable method as the catheter tip during injection usually moves out of the scanning plane whereby part of the catheter can be misinterpreted as the tip. Marking of the catheter tip with a material of different acoustic properties acting as a passive reflector was promising in an in vitro experiments, but unsatisfactory in vivo. This is because of the numerous echoes from the already-mentioned cardiac structures or spurious echoes which obscure the image of the tip reflector.

We have solved the problem of identification of the catheter tip by mounting a cylindrical miniature transducer unit and by the use of associate electronics. The catheter transducer can act in an active or passive mode. In the active system an external pulse generator connected to the catheter transducer induces ultrasonic pulses which are picked up by the scanner transducer. These appear on the 2-dimensional echocardiographic image as a bright line always crossing the catheter transducer. The main advantages of this system are simplicity and independence of the scanner. Its disadvantages are the introduction of relatively high voltages (up to 10 V) into the heart (necessitating special safety insulation) and the lack of depth resolution.

In the passive system the catheter transducer acts as a receiver of the ultrasound pulses from the external transducer. The principle of operation is illustrated in Fig. 4. The catheter transducer is

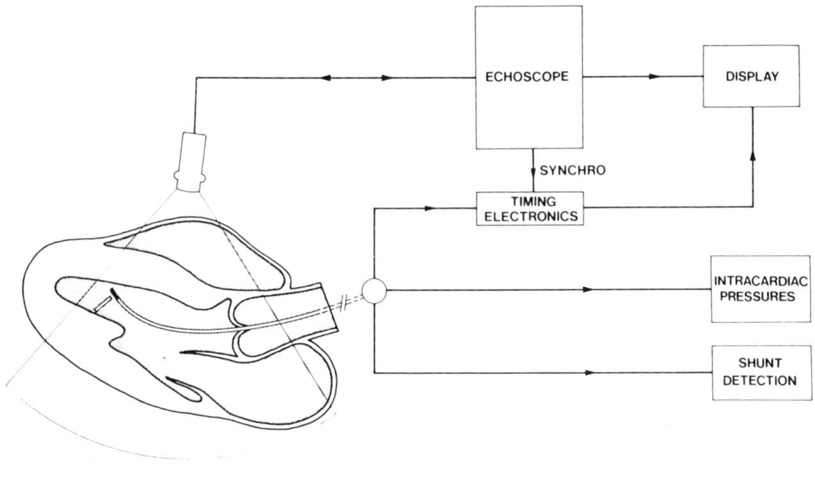

Fig. 4 Passive system for marking of the catheter
The catheter transducer acts as a reciever of the ultrasound pulses from the external transducer. Thereby the catheter tip is indicated by a short line.

triggered by ultrasound pulses from the scanner transducer and the voltage generated is transmitted to the timing electronics where it can be amplified and used for timing. The time between ultrasound transmission from the scanner transducer and detection by the catheter transducer must be doubled in order to position the marker signal correctly. As a result, a well-defined blinking marker adjacent to the catheter tip can be seen on the 2-dimensional echocardiographic image. The blinking marker can be easily differentiated from the cardiac structures and is visible at any gain setting. The passive system has the advantages that it does not introduce electrical pulses into the heart, it has the best marker properties and a good axial and lateral resolution. Its only disadvantage is scanner dependence such that the timing electronics input and output must be differently designed for different scanners.

The efficacy of the prototype system was tested in a water-bath, in cadaveric hearts and in beating dog hearts. In all instances the blinking marker of the catheter tip was easily identified and correctly positioned. With this system it seems that echocardiography can be used not only for obtaining unique morphologic data but also for additional data on intracardiac pressures and oxymetric data for the calculation of intracardiac shunts. Angiography may be performed using indifferent echo-contrast. The same system can be used in guiding and assessing myocardial perfusion studies.

Our previous animal study with a home-made prototype system showed the feasibility of the procedure. Recently, first catheters and pacing leads for human use have been designed. Our first clinical experience using such device will be presented.

Utilizing standard 2-dimensional echocardiographic transducer approaches a blinking signal adjacent to the catheter or lead tip can be seen in different planes allowing its precise positioning within cardiac cavities. Except in cardiac cavities the catheter signal can be followed through abdominal aorta, aortic arch, ascending aorta and superior and inferior vena cava. (Figs. 5,6,7).

The advantages of echo guided cardiac catheterization over conventional X-ray guided catheterization are the avoidance of ionising radiation, as well as of the toxic and hemodynamic effects of iodine contrast medium, better spatial anatomy due to the multiple sectional planes which allow for precise positioning of catheter tip, and finally the fact that this method is considerably

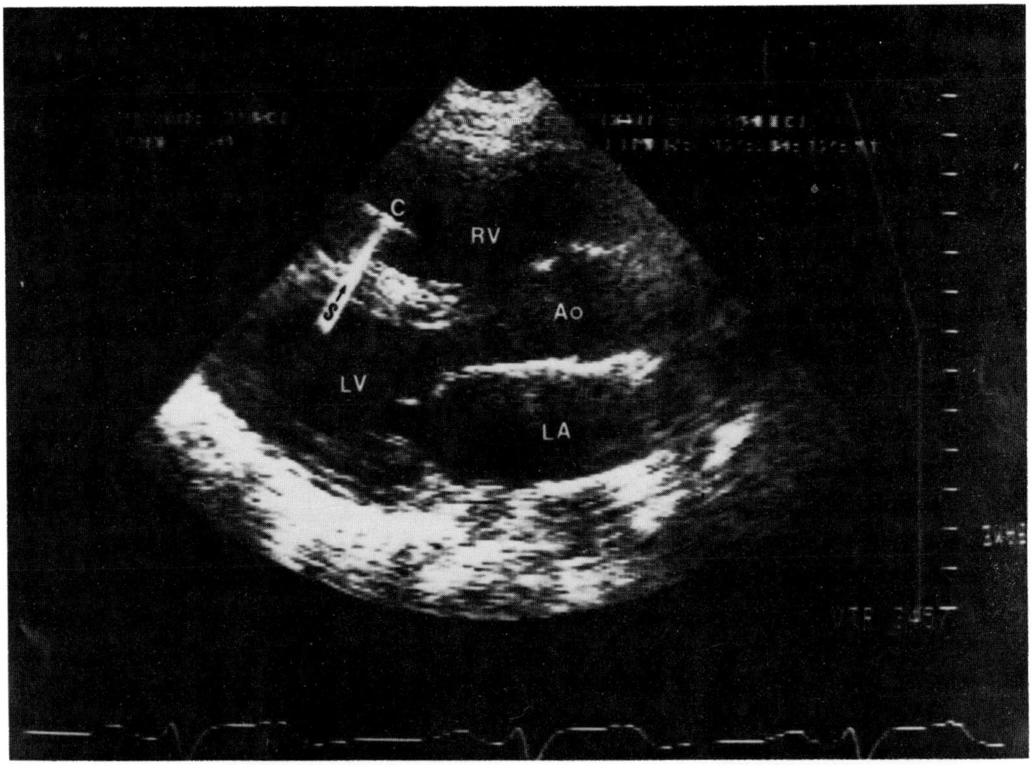

Fig. 5 Long axis section with ortogonally sected catheter (C) tip indicated by the signal (S)

less expensive, allowing its use in smaller centers. Disadvantages are lack of coronary angiography and poor images in some patients with a small "echo-window".

It seems likely that after a clinical trial the method can become a procedure for complete cardiac diagnosis; in the majority of patients it can possibly replace X-ray guided cardiac catheterization.

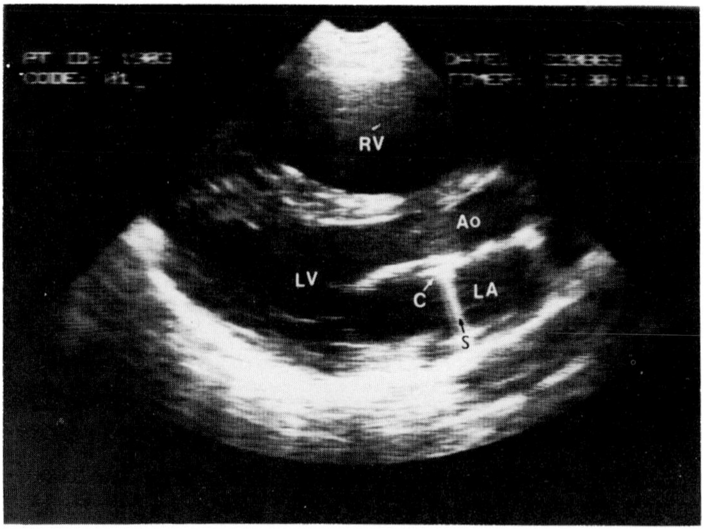

Fig. 6 In patient with atrial septal defect the catheter (C) has passed through the defect from right atrium to the left atrium as indicated by the signal (S).

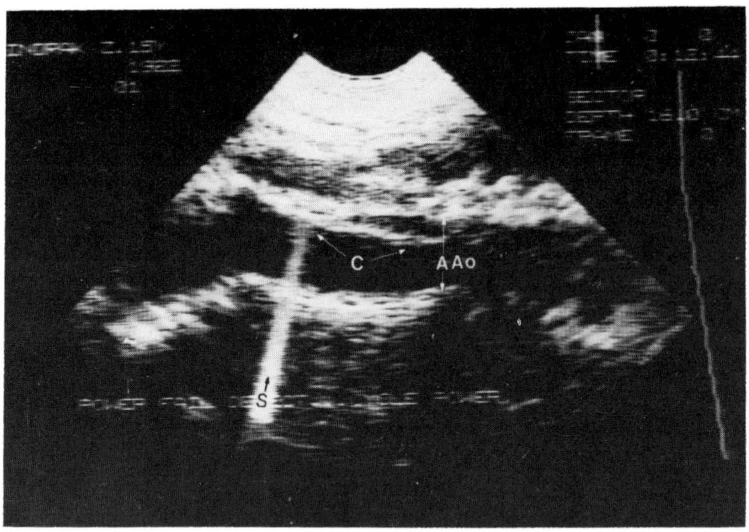

Fig. 7 The catheter (C) is imaged in abdominal aorta (AAo). Its tip is indicated by the signal (S).

ULTRASONICALLY GUIDED INTRODUCTION OF PACING AND ELECTROPHYSIOLOGIC ELECTRODES

Recently, we have used the passive system for marking the tip of pacemaker and electrophysiologic electrodes. It allows electrode introduction and precise positioning under echo guidance. It may also be used for better diagnosis of acute and chronic pacing system malfunction. Precise diagnosis of dislodgement, microdislodgement and myocardial perforation is possible. The M- mode technique has been found to be superior for the identification of electrode microdislodgement.

A pacemaker has been adapted for telemetry of pulses from the electrode transducer, allowing for additional electronic control. Thus, non-invasive discrimination between lead fracture (X-ray invisible) and pulse generator failure in cases of loss of pacing pulse is possible. As high frequency control of the echo signal is more sensitive on lead impedance alternation, the insulation break detection in early phase is possible.

Marking electrophysiologic electrodes by the passive system provides exact placement of the His electrode, endocardial mapping, and perhaps in the near future percutaneous catheter ablative therapy.

REFERENCES

1. Cikes I (1983) Interventional echocardiography. In: 5th Symposium on Echocardiology. Rotterdam, Abstracts p 38

2. Cikeš I, Ernst A, Breyer B (1983) Interventional echocardiography, 3rd International Congress on Interventional Ultrasound. Copenhagen, Abstracts p 102

3. Cikeš I, Ernst A (1983) New aspects of echocardiography for the diagnosis and treatment of pericardial disease. In: Roelandt J (ed) The practice of M-mode and two-dimensional echocardiography. The Hague, Boston, London:Martinus Nijhoff Publishers, 141

4. Cikes I, Breyer B, Ernst A, Custovič F (1984) Cardiac catheterization guided by ultrasound, JACC, 3:564

5. Cikes I (1984) Echocardiography to guide interventions, 4th International Congress on Echocardiology, Verona, Abstracts p 35

6. Hanraht P, Bleifeld W, Souquet J (eds) (1982) Cardiovascular diagnosis by ultrasound. Transesophageal, computerized, contrast Doppler echocardiography. The Hague, Boston,London: Martinus Nijhoff Publishers.

7. Cikeš I (1982) New echocardiographic possibilities in the etiological diagnosis and therapy of pericardial diseases. In: Hanrath P, Bleifeld W, Souquet J (eds) Cardiovascular diagnosis by ultrasound. The Hague, Boston, London: Martinus Nijhoff

Publishers, 188

8. Roelandt J (1983) In: Roelandt J (ed) The practice of M-mode and two-dimensional echocardiography. The Hague, Boston, London: Martinus Nijhoff Publishers

9. Cikes I, Breyer B (1983) Complete cardiac catheterization guided by ultrasound. Eur Heart J, 4 (suppl E):21

10. Mortensen SA, Egeblad H (1983) Endomyocardial biopsy guided by cross-sectional echocardiography. Br Heart J, 50:246

11. Breyer B, Cikes I (1984) Ultrasonically marked catheter - a method for positive echographic catheter position identification. Med Biol Eng Comput, 22:268

12. Cikeš I, Breyer B, Ernst A, Custović F (1985) Interventional echocardiography. In: Holm HH, Kristensen JK (eds) Interventional Ultrasound. Copenhagen, Munksgaard, 160

Recent advances in ultrasound diagnosis 5. A. Kurjak, G. Kossoff, eds.

INTERVENTIONAL ULTRASOUND IN UROLOGY

HANS HENRIK HOLM

Department of Ultrasound, Herlev Hospital, University of Copenhagen, DK-273o Herlev, Denmark.

It is universally recognized that ultrasound has changed the speciality of obstetrics fundamentally because of the tremendous amount of new information which quite easily is provided by this technique.

However, I think it is fair to postulate that at present a similar development is taken place in urology. In other words that the urological speciality is changing considerably under the influence of diagnostic and therapeutic (or interventional) ultrasound.

Traditionally the I.V.P. and the cystoscope are considered the most important diagnostic tools in urology. Undoubtedly, I.V.P. is still quite necessary e.g. in the diagnosis of stones in the ureter and small pelvic papillomas etc. Likewise, cystoscopy is of course quite indispensable e.g. in diagnosis and treatment of bladder tumors.

However, the constant refinement of dynamic ultrasound scanners has made the technique highly competitive with conventional x-rays in several areas such as in evaluation of hydronephrosis and renal masses - and obviously superior in other areas as e.g. in perirenal collections and in the detection of bladder tumors.

Furthermore, certain structures such as the prostate and the testes which previously could not be visualized at all, can now be demonstrated beautifully by ultrasound.

Special equipment designed for the urologist are available at the market e.g. transurethral- and transrectal scanners.

They provide excellent images of the bladder, prostate and seminal vesicles facilitating detection and staging of neoplastic diseases in these organs.

Although regular control cystoscopy is necessary in the majority of bladder tumor patients, abdominal ultrasound + urine cytology can replace cystoscopy in a significant number of low malignant tumors.

Today other techniques such as CT and MR providing beautiful sectional images compete with ultrasound.

However, usually after a while the urologist becomes accustomed to the nature and the peculiarity of the ultrasound image.

When at the same time he realizes that ultrasound usually provides the same amount of information and understands the many advantages of ultrasound such as availability, convenience, mobility, cost, dynamic imaging, unlimited number of plans etc. ultrasound will often become his favorite diagnostic tool. It will probably replace I.V.P. in many of its traditional areas e.g. the patient with hematuria, with chronic urinary infection, with infravesical obstruction, palpable masses etc. etc.

One very important additional use in urology is interventional ultrasound.[1]

Interventional ultrasound has an important role to play in the upper as well as in the lower urinary tract.

Thus, ultrasonically guided puncture has numerous applications in the kidney. E.g. ordinary large bore biopsies in the evaluation of acute or chronic nephrological diseases are best performed under ultrasonic guidance, which is quite independant of renal function. A longitudinal scan in the prone position is preferable. The biopsy is taken from the lower pole using a Silvermann or a True-cut needle.

In our institution the only problem is whether the nephrologist or the ultrosonologist shall perform the biopsy.

Focal renal lesions are another obvious area for interventional ultrasound. Modern ultrasound equipment can in the large majority of cases where I.V.P. has disclosed a spaceoccupying lesion - quite reliably distinguish between a harmless cyst and a solid tumor.

It is well known, however, that a small per cent of cystic renal lesions is malignant - probably approximately 1%. The very first renal cyst we punctured many years ago was ultrasonically and arteriographically a typical large cyst and the cyst fluid was clear when aspirated. The fluid, however, contained tumorcells. The cyst was resected and turned out to have a thin layer of tumorcells in the whole circumference. The patient later died of lung metastases. This is an extremely rare tumor type and despite we have punctured many hundreds renal cysts -

almost all we have seen - since then we have seen anything similar.

We feel now that it is unnecessary to puncture completely asymptomatic, ultrasonically quite typical renal cysts. If there is the slightest suspicion, however, we do an ultrasonically guided puncture, empty the cyst completely, and send the fluid for cytology and cholesterol determination which according to the literature is the most sensitive test for malignancy.

If there is any doubt whether a small central fluid collection is a calyx cyst or a renal cyst a few drops of the fluid on a "stix" will reveal its nature since only a cyst will normally contain protein and sugar.

The true nature of a solid renal mass or of a suspicious area can often be disclosed by a guided fine needle biopsy.

The difficulties with renal cytology especially the not insignificant number of false positives have previously been mentioned.

At present the most promising biopsy approach in solid renal masses seems to be a o.8 mm (21 gauge) histological biopsy (sure-cut type). Sufficient material is with this technique obtained in the large majority of cases and the very unpleasant false positives are avoided.

Unless embolization of the tumor is found indicated the preoperative evaluation of the renal tumor patient can usually be reduced to ultrasonic scanning including biopsy and a renogram.

For the urologist fine needle biopsies of suspected liver metastases or enlarged retroperitoneal lymph nodes is important in the management of patients with neoplastic disease in the kidney, bladder, prostata and testes.

The first intraabdominal abscess treated percutaneously by ultrasonically guided puncture was a renal abscess. It was done in our laboratory and the outcome was quite succesful.

Peroperative ultrasound - sometimes involving guided puncture - has become increasingly popular especially in liver surgery, in vascular surgery and in neurosurgery.

The technique has also proved increasingly useful in renal surgery especially in the localization of renal stone fragments thereby facilitating their removal considerably.

However, since conventional renal stone surgery (because of the introduction of percutaneous techniques) has become more or less obsolete during the last few years peroperative renal ultrasound is only used infrequently.

Percutaneous access to the renal pelvis is, on the other hand, being used more and more to drain hydro- or pyonephrosis as well as for endoscopic renal surgery for renal stones, for certain pelvic tumors and for selected cases of ureteropelvic junction obstruction.

When a hydronephrosis has been diagnosed either by ultrasound or by some other imaging modality, the need for a nephrostomy may arise. If there is only need for a temporary nephrostomy with an expected drainage time of a few days or antegrad pyelography is going to be performed a "pig-tail catheter" is well suited. A needle with stylet is placed inside the "pig-tail catheter", which is advanced guided by ultrasound into the renal pelvis. When the tip of the needle is seen in place, the stylet is removed and when urine escapes the needle is withdrawn leaving the curled tipcatheter in place.

However, in many cases there is a need for a more permanent nephrostomy as e.g. in renal obstruction due to recurrence of a cervix carcinoma.

Although, fixed to the skin the "pig-tail catheter" has the disadvantage of slipping out unintended in many cases, requiring re-nephrostomy.

To solve this problem we developed a balloon catheter nephrostomy set, which due to the balloon has an internal fixation. The set consists of a 1.2 mm (18 gauge) puncture needle with stylet, a Lunderquist PE 9o guidewire with a soft tip, 3 plastic dilators sized from 8 F to 14 F and a lo F silicone balloon catheter with a hole in its tip. After puncture of the collecting system in local anaesthetics the guidewire is inserted and the needle removed. After subsequent dilatation with the 3 plastic dilators the balloon catheter is inserted and the balloon inflated whereupon the guidewire is removed. The catheter is also sutured to the skin.

The nephrostomy system has been used in 52 consecutive attempts during a period of 18 months.

The nephrostomy was succesful in 51 cases.

It failed in one young male patient with congenital bilateral hydronephrosis. The kidney parenchyma had a consistenc like leather and we were not able to dilate a tract. The hydronephroses were drained with pig-tail catheters and werc later operated upon.

The nephrostomies were preserved from 2 to 15o days. In some cases the kidney were operated upon after a few days and in some cases fluoroscopic stentning was tried after 3-4 days of drainage.

However, what it worth noticing is that none of the balloon catheters slipped out unintended earlier than 27 days after the nephrostomy. This means that once a balloon catheter has been placed the rate of the inconvenient re-nephrostomies is reduced significantly.

When endoscopic renal surgery is carried out a reasonably sized tract to an appropriate part of the pelviocalyceal system has to be established.

To reduce the damage to the renal parenchyma and also to avoid the larger vessels - especially the interlobar arteries - access via a calyx is clearly preferable.

To increase the space between the 12th rib and the iliac crest and to immobilize the kidney we find it advantageous to elevate the renal region in question - on the patient in the prone position - with a pillow. To avoid with certainty transpleural puncture it is generally recommendable to do the puncture below the 12th rib or in the lower most intercostal space.

Because of the anatomical condition just mentioned, the calyx best suited for puncture is the lower major calyx via a minor calyx located posteriorly. Even then a rather cephalad puncture direction is necessary. To enter the major calyx in its longitudinal direction a puncture site approximately 15 cm lateral for the midline is in most cases appropriate.

How ideal an access through the lower calyx is depends of course of the location and type of pathology but it is remarcable how well most of the pelviocalyceal system can be reached via this approach even with a rigid nephroscope. This is because of the considerable mobility of the kidney. Other calyces can of course be punctured if necessary.

An important prerequisite for the subsequent dilatation and endoscope insertion is a correct needle placement.

How can this best be accomplished?

When the calyceal system is hydronephrotic the puncture generally presents no problem. When it is non-dilated it may be difficult.

At least three possibilities are available:

1. X-ray fluoroscopy guided by an intravenous pyelogram. Although x-ray in two plans in principle is to be preferred this is in practive too cumbersome to work with. A drawback using this technique may be that the continuous excretion of contrast may obscure stone fragments during the following stone removal.

2. X-ray fluoroscopy guided by retrograde pyelography through a ureteric catheter is another possibility. Advantages are that contrast can be injected whenever required and that the catheter hopefully prevents that stone fragments escape into the ureter. A drawback is the time required for the cystoscopy. In both cases one dimension is missing during the needle insertion.

3. The third possibility is an ultrasonically guided puncture of the calyx. The advantage is that since the needle is inserted along a predetermined needlepath in the image plan, only one plan is needed to completely identify the ideal needlepath. Another advantage is that the amount of ionizing radiation is reduced. A drawback is that the needle tip echo and a non-dilated calyx may be difficult to see in very heavy patients.

A stone is definitely visible when it is 5 mm or more and shows up as a strong echo reflection with posterior shadowing.

Ideally a hydronephrosis has each calyx group visible.

To dilate the collecting system 1-2 liter of glucose is administered i.v. together with 4o mg of lasix. A bladder catheter is inserted but we do not use a ureteral catheter.

A sterilized scanner is used for the puncture of the collecting system which is almost always clearly visible after hydration.

The scanner is moved and tilted until the punctureline on the monitor coincides with the desired needle path right into the calyx.

When the needle tip echo is in the collecting system and urine hopefully appears from the needle the soft tip guidewire is inserted.

After initial dilatation with 3 small plastic dilators a safety guidewire is also inserted. Contrast is injected and correct position of the two guidewires is ascertained.

The dilatation of the tract is either performed with Storz's telescope dilators or more often with Cook's plastic dilators.

The insertion of each dilator is ensured fluoroscopically.

A plastic sheath is then inserted over the last dilator - usually Ch. no. 3o.

The dilator is removed.

The nephroscope is then inserted and it is attempted to remove the stone in one piece. If the stone is too large to be removed in one piece an ultrasound stone disintegrator is used.

A balloon catheter is finally left in place for one day unless bleeding or lesion of the renal pelvis indicates prolonged drainage.

Together with the Rigshospital we have treated 125 patients according to these principles.

We do not necessarily reduce operation time but reduce postoperative hospitalization to an average of 4 days, and reduce convalescence time and postoperative pain considerably.

Interventional ultrasound does not play a prominent role in the urinary bladder although it can be used as a guide in suprapubic puncture and in puncturing balloon catheters which cannot be emptied the usual way.

Puncture guided by transrectal scanning - transverse or longitudinal - plays on the other hand an increasingly important role.

It is well recognized that transrectal scanning is highly reliable in the diagnosis of prostatic cancer if the prostatic capsule is penetrated and even slight extraprostatic tumorgrowth is present.

It is, however, also known that it is difficult to diagnose cancer based upon the internal echopattern alone.

A special biopsy technique has therefore been developed based on which tissue samples can be obtained precisely from predetermined suspicious areas on the transrectal prostatic scan.

This has proved most useful in dayly clinical practice and also to gain knowledge about the meaning of the ultrasound image.

The same technique allows also for precise needling of the seminal vesicles. Thereby e.g. an abscess in one of these organs can be emptied.

Based upon the pioneer work by Whitmore, Hilaris and Grabstald[2] on I^{125} seed implantation in prostatic cancer we have at the departments of Urology, Ultrasound and Oncology at the Herlev

Hospital made an attempt to develope a method for seed implantation in the prostate less traumatic, time consuming and expensive than the conventional surgical one - and hopefully also more precise.[3]

When suspicion of prostatic cancer has arisen transrectal ultrasonic scanning of the prostate is carried out to exclude extracapsular tumorgrowth - as well as a guided microcore biopsy from the ultrasonically suspicious area - if any.

Provided the ultrasound examination demonstrates that no extracapsular tumorgrowth is present and the biopsy shows a poorly or medium differentiated cancer the following examinations are carried out to demonstrate metastatic disease or the localized nature of the cancer:

Ultrasonic scanning of the liver and retroperitoneum,

X-ray of thorax,

Bone scintigraphy and

Extraperitoneal pelvioscopy as described by Hald and Rasmussen.[4]

The presence of lymph node metastases is obviously important for the actual patient's prognosis. However, it does not seem to be likely that a lymphadenectomy, which necessitates an open operation, improves the prognosis. This to us justifies the use of the new technique although the evaluation of the lymph nodes probably is somewhat less precise than with an open operation.

When seed implantation has been decided upon a series of prostatic scans spaced by ½ cm is produced with the patient in the lithotomy position and the rectal scanner in a fixture.

By outlining each prostatic section by a lightpen the computer in the scanner calculates the volume of the gland which is used as a baseline study.

On the basis of the same series of scans the physicist calculates the seed distribution and orders the necessary number of seeds from the manufacturer.

When the seeds have arrived they are loaded together with cromic catgut spacers in a number of 1.3 mm needles according to the precalculated treatment program and the needles are sterilized.

In spinal anaesthesia the patient is placed in exactly the same position as during the initial planning procedure. The rectal scanner - mounted with a special multichannel puncture attachment - is again mounted in the fixture and brought in correct position.

Guided by the ultrasonic scan each needle, containing from 1 to 6 seeds and spacers is now inserted through the appropriate channel into the prostate.

When a strong echo on the scan indicates that the needle tip is in the correct location the seeds and spacers are released by withdrawing the needle while a stylet keeps the content of the needle in place in the prostate. The needles are inserted without paying attention to the urethra.

The result of the seed implantation can be demonstrated on a series of ultrasound scans of the prostate where the seeds show up as strong echoreflections and on x-ray.

The minimum tumordose from the seeds is 16o Gy.

The patient is usually discharged from the hospital the following day.

One month following the implantation the patient receives 4o Gy in a series of external irradiations on the pelvic region including the prostate.

The patients are followed up according to a protocol which includes transrectal scan of the prostate including volume determination every third and later every sixth month as well as prostatic biopsies one, two and three years after the treatment.

We have carried this procedure out for approximately two years. During which period lo patients with poorly to medium differentiated prostatic cancers have had 17-61 seeds implanted using 12-26 punctures. From the x-rays it appeared that the seeds were correctly and evenly distributed. Four of the patients passed a few seeds during the subsequent micturitions.

In all the 9 patients in whom we had an opportunity to carry out repeated volume determinations of the prostate a significant reduction in prostatic volume was found following the seed implantation.

In the 4 patients who had a control biopsy of the prostate performed approximately one year later, fibrosis but no tumor tissue was found. In one of the patients, however, a biopsy after lo months still revealed some areas with cancer. 3 patients developed distant metastases.

The following early complications developed during the observation period:

There were no bleeding or hematoma formation.

Three patients became more infravesically obstructed than before the implantation and in one case transurethral resection was necessary. 3 got a temporary urinary tract infection succesfully treated with antibiotics. One became slightly incontinent. Two patients complained of reduced potency and one of moderate diarrhoea but this both symptoms diminished after completion of the external radiation.

The patient material is too small to draw any firm conclusions. However, the complication rate seems to be low and the preliminary results suggest that it is possible in the majority of cases to control the local cancergrowth.

REFERENCES

1. Holm HH, Kristensen JK (1985) (eds) Interventional Ultrasound. Munksgaard, Copenhagen
2. Hilaris BS (1975) (eds) Handbook of Interstitial Brachytherapy. Publishing Sciences Group, Inc., Acton, Massachusetts
3. Holm HH, Gammelgaard J (1981) J Urol 125:385
4. Hald T, Rasmussen F (198o) J Urol 125:245

Recent advances in ultrasound diagnosis 5. A. Kurjak, G. Kossoff, eds.

INTERVENTIONAL ULTRASOUND IN UROLOGIC THERAPY

MARJAN RADEJ
Department of Urology, General Hospital "Dr.Josip Kajfeš" Zagreb, Yugoslavia.

Recent advances in ultrasound and uroradiology have markedly broadened the scope of the combined team of the urologic surgeon and uroradiologist. The new concepts have revolutionized the traditional urologic approaches to such entities such as obstructive uropathy, renal masses, renovascular hypertension, urolithiasis and the staging of urologic cancers. Interventional ultrasound procedures do not represent a threat to traditional urologic surgery. They should be viewed as a reafirement of fundamental concepts in urology, saving formal surgery for these patients, who cannot be managed by less agressive means. Percutaneous catheterization under the ultrasonic guidance of the needle of the biliary tree, renal collecting system and cavities in various areas of the body has become routine in many centers.

The dilated kidney hole system could be easy detected by the ultrasonic exploration. This fact is the ground for the most important ultrasonic interventional procedure - the percutaneous insertion of catheters into the renal pelvis. It enables us to perform the other procedures, for instance the dilatation of the new obtained channel that gives the possibility for percutaneous lithotripsy, biopsy of renal tumors, instilation of drugs, or dilatation of ureteral strictures (Fig. 1).

The currently available nephrostomy sets consist of a flexible guide wire, progressive dilators and pigtail catheter. The wire provides guidance for dilators and the catheter into the renal pelvis. Several dilators are used, depending on the diameter of the catheter to be inserted into the pyelocaliceal system. The dilators are inserted and removed over the guide wire until the tract is large enough to allow passage of the nephtostomy catheter.

The tools used for this procedure include B-mode ultrasonography to locate the depth and direction of the dilated collecting system. The skin is infiltrated with a local anesthetic and incised a few mm at the puncture site. The puncture is performed with a 3 part needle (outer canula and inner beveled needle with stylet). It is made below the 12th rib. The needle is angled 45 degrees to the table top while being directed towards the cortex.

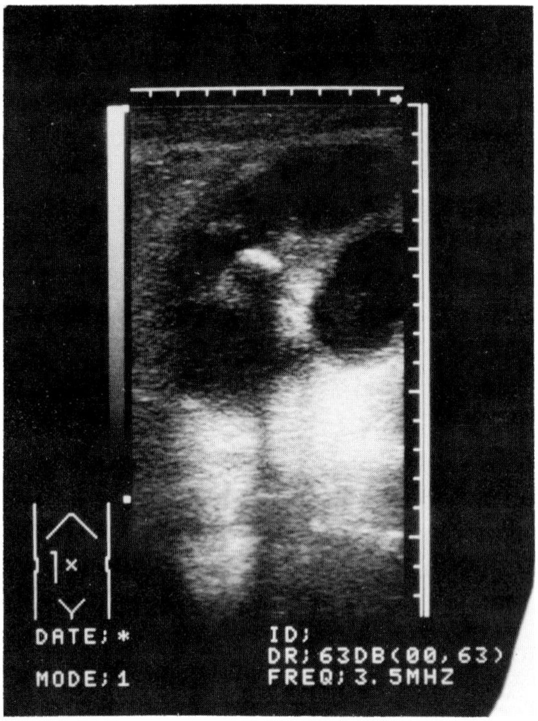

Fig. 1. Ultrasonic presentation of hydronephrosis with stone.

It is important to emphasize that the needle should pass through the cortex. This way, good support for advancement of the dilators and catheter is possible, while avoiding the major vessels at the hilus. It is advisable to puncture the kidney with a 23 gauge Chiba needle. A syringe is connected with the fine needle and is held under constant negative pressure. Once the needle tip enters the renal cavity, urine flows into the syringe. It is easy to place the guide wire through the needle into the pelvis. The best result is obtained if it is possible to introduce the guide wire into the proximal part of ureter.

This technique is applicable to children including neonates too. General anesthesis is usually employed to avoid the need for infiltration of local anesthetic agents and to allow an operation to proceed immediately so that obstruction could be confirmed. Spiral needle of 20 or 22 gauge is advanced through the renal angle just below the 12th rib. A respiratory swing of the needle indicates that contact has been made with the renal substance. If in the operating theatre the x-ray control is available, it is possible to inject contrast media (Hypaque 25%). The further technical procedure is the same as for adults.

Until recently, the indications for percutaneous nephrostomy were limited for the patients requiring temporary drainage, that is: 1) postoperative obstruction or extravasation 2) ureteral obstruction secondary to carcinoma responsive to chemotherapy or radiotherapy, 3) preoperative stabilization before relief of obstruction caused by ureteral calculus in patients with solytary kidneys or sepsis and 4) preoperative evaluation of renal function and degree of obstruction.

Improved methodology and equipment have expanded this significant list to include the following: 1) irrigation of dissolveable stones through the nephrostomy, 2) placement of permanent nephrostomy and 3) the use of the nephrostomy tract as a conduit to the collecting system for stone manipulation, biopsies and placement of ureteral stents. (Figs. 1 and 2).

The only absolute contraindication of percutaneous nephrostomy is a significant bleeding diathesis.

It is difficult to say whether the antegrade pyeography will substitute the retrograde ureteral catheterization or not. The major disadvantages of ureteral catheterization are the obstruction may reocur after catheter removal, and infection may be introduced. The percutaneous nephrostomy offers the advantages of remaining in situ and being easily clamped temporarily, while giving the patients a trial of spontaneous stone passage. Today it is possible to manage succsessfully even the large infected obstructing stones in eldery patients, when immediate surgery is not feasible. The complications reported at the application of percutaneous nephrostomy have included 1-2 per cent infection, 1-2 per cent hemorrhage and 1 per cent urine leakege. It is obvious that the complications rate will be higher at the beginning of the interventions, and will be deminished with the increasing experience.

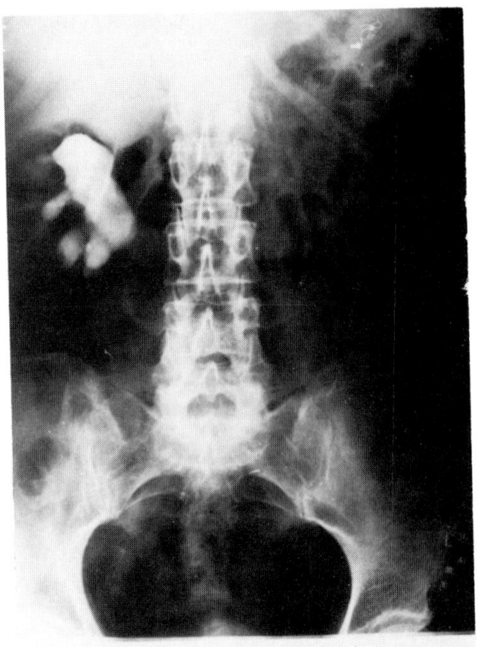

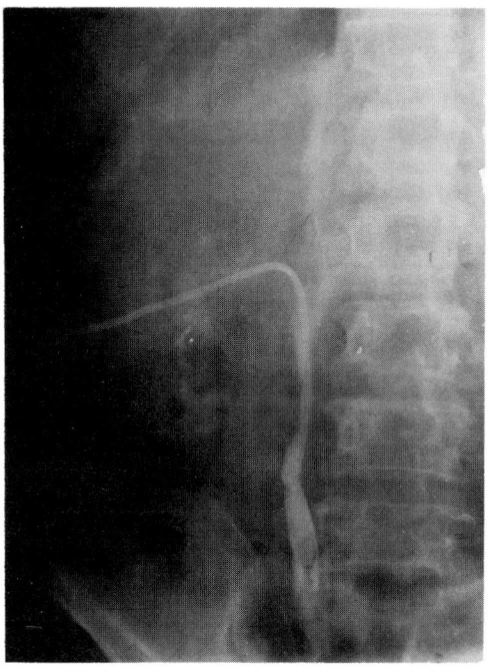

Figs. 2.and 3. Malignant ureteral obstruction of the single right kidney (left) and percutaneous nephrostomy (right)

Percutaneous removal of renal stones in becoming an established procedure, especially for stones lying free in the renal pelvis. However, some renal stones, particulary caliceal stones, are less accessible, and require special techniques for removal. The site of entry into the kidney is important, particulary when percutaneous nephrostomy for the removal of caliceal stones is performed. The flank should be punctered posterolaterally, and the collecting system should be entered through the lateral aspect of the renal parenchyma. It is useful to insert the second safety guide wire or catheter as a precaution against loss of access during the manipulation. The best is to enter the collecting system just medial to the stone. Every effort should be made to place the puncture below the 12th rib otherwise we could face intrathoracal complications (pneumothorax, hydrothorax). Previously we should insert an ureter into the renal pelvis to avoid ureteral obstruction by stone fragments, and to enable filling or empting the pelvis with second source of water. Dilators 5 F to 24 F are passed over the guide wire beyond the stone. After that procedure, it is simple to enter the operating sheath with optical system and ultrasonic lithotrite. After visualization of the stone the lithotrite should be gently pressed to it, and the lithotripsy starts. The mechanic vibrational energy, produced within the ultrasonic transducer, is transferred through a thin metal tube -the ultrasonic probe- to the working or oscillating tip located at the distal end of the probe. These oscillations fragmented the stone, and detritus is washed out by low pressure of irrigated liquid. The small particle of stones can be extracted by forceps.

Today are manufactured the fleksible nephro and ureteroscopes which enable the accurate way to the caliceal and ureteral stones.

After the stone is removed, the 2o F nephrostomy tube should be placed into the percutaneous channel for 3-4 days. It enables the drainage and irrigation of the collecting system preventing the postoperative bleeding too.

There is no doubt that the patients will choose least invasive surgery if possible. They will not allow to be disturbed by a long classical surgical procedures, if they can be treated with the same results and leave the hospitale in a few days.(Fig. 4).

The second noninvasive method of stone destruction by shock waves, also seems not to be competitive to the ultrasonic destruction. The main advantage of the latter method is the possibility to remove completely the collecting system from stone detritus by washing out through the percutaneous tube. It also facilitates the renewal of the procedure in a few days after the first failure. The removal of renal calculi by open surgical intervention (stag-horne stones) often entails a belance between the duration of the search and degree of tissue manipulation and dissection.

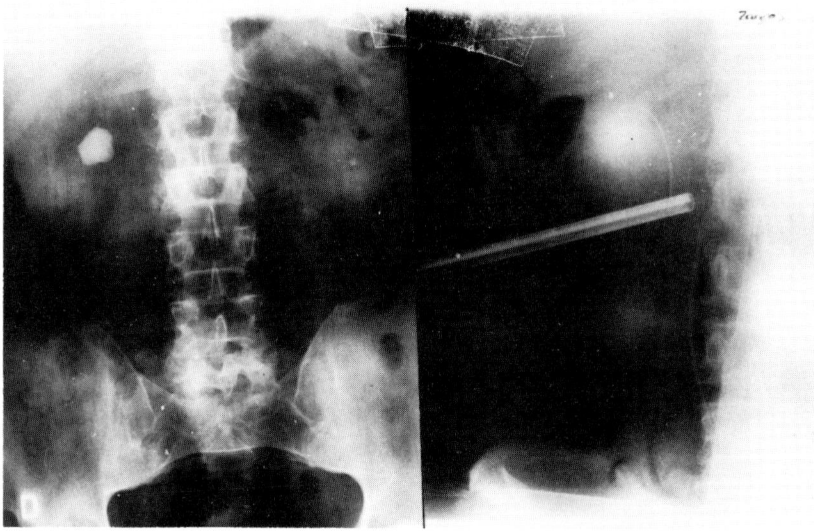

Fig. 4. Stone in the right kidney (left).Percutaneous stone destru ction by ultrasonic probe (right).

The latter equates with a greater potential for renal parenchymal damage and increased morbidity. Surgical ultrasonografy offers a better detection of intrarenal stones. The 2-dimensional real time B-mode ultrasound imaging in kidney detects the stone at less than 3 cm below the tissue surface by the use of high frequency instruments (7,5 to lo m Hz frequency range). By exploration of the kidney by a Doppler device the blood vessels around the stone can be located, and the site of smoll incision at the most convenient place, can be chosen.

Stone dissolution was an ideal goal for centuries in urology. During the last 2 decades there have been numerous reports on successful dissolution of uric acid calculi. Since the solubility of uric acid increases dramatically with a modest increase in urinary pH, it is not surprising that many authors have reported that uric acid stones can be dissolved by the peroral drugs balancing the urine pH betwen 6,5 to 7.o. But using the percutaneous nephrostomy and irrigating the renal pelvis and stone by the application of sodium chloride pH 7,6 the stone can be dissoluted in less lo days.

More interesting struvite stones represent the more dificult problem, and their connection with inflammation and recurency is one of the greatest problem in urology. Fortunatelly the recent reports suggest the optimistic possibilities, and some authors have reported a satisfectory results using the lo per cent solution of hemiacidrine through the percutaneous renal tube. It is only important to keep the intrarenal pressure of irrigation solution under the pressure of 25 cm water.

The similar results have been obtained in the attempt to dissolute the cystine calculi using the N - acetylcisteine.

The traditional management of renal abscess is either nephrectomy or open surgical drainage. In the recent urologic literature the successful treatment of 6 patients by a combination of antibiotic therapy and percutaneous drainage, was described.

The same results are described in many reports concerning the treatment of the solitary renal cysts. It is easy to locate the cyst by the ultrasound and to puncture its content. After the cytologic examination one can decide about the indication for surgery. In the most cases the percutaneous procedure completes the treatment.

In our hospital we have performed 172 percutaneous interventions on the kidney. lol ultrasonic litothripsy, 25 ultrasonically guided punctions of renal cysts and 46 percutaneous nephrostomies in various indications, mostly as an act in emergency. By the high rate of success with a minimum number of complications we have beeb also convinced of a great value of this new therapeutic methods in urology.

BIBLIOGRAPHY

1. Bean,W.J.: Renal Cysts: Treatment with Alcohol.Diagnostic Radiology, 2:33o, 1981.

2. Burns, J.R.,Gauthier,J.F., Finlayson, B.: Dissolution Kinetics of Uric Acid Calculi.J.Urol., 131:7o8, 1984.

3. Burns, J.R., Gauthier, J.F.: Prevention of Urinary Catheter Incrustations By Acetohydroxamic Acid. J. Urol., 132:455, 1985.

4. Chan, J.C.M., Brewer, W.H., Still, W.J.: Renal Biopsies Under Ultrasound Guidance: loo Consecutive Biopsies in Children. J. Urol., 129:lo3, 1983.

5. Chaussy, C., Schmiedt, E., Jocham, D., Brendel, W.,Forssmann, B., Walther, V.: First Clinical experience with exracorporeally induced destruction of kidney Stones By Shockwaves. J.Urol., 127:417, 1982.

6. Clayman, R.V., Hunter,D., Surya, V., Castaneda-Zuniga,W.R., Amplatz, D., Lange, P.H.: Percutaneous Intrarenal Electrosurgery. J.Urol., 131:864, 1984.

7. Clayman, R.V., Surya,V., Castaneda-Zuniga, W.R., Miller, R.P., Lange, P.H.: Percutaneous Nephrolithotomy with Mazzariello-Caprini Forceps. J. Urol., 129ß1213, 1983.

8. Clayman,R.V., Surya, V., Hunter, D.,Castaneda-Zuniga, W.R., Miller, R.P., Coleman, C., Amplatz, D., Lange,P.H.: Renal Vascular Complications Associated With Percutaneous Removal of Renal Calculi. J. Urol., 132:228, 1984.

9. Clayman,R.V., Surya, V., Miler,R.P., Castaneda-Zuniga, W.R., Smith,A.D., Hunter, D.H., Amplatz, D., Lange,P.H.: Percutaneous Nephrolythotomy: Extraction of Renal and Ureteral Calculi From loo Patients. J. Urol., 131:868, 1984.

lo. Dretler,S.Pl., Pfister,R.C., Newhouse, J.H.,Priem, JR.E.L.: Percutaneous Catheter Dissolution of Cystine Calculi.J. Urol., 131:216, 1984.

11. Dretler,S.P., Pfister,R.C.: Primary Dissolution Therapy of Struvite Calculi.J. Urol., 131:861, 1984.

12. Elder,J.S., Gibbons, R.P., Bush, W.H.: Ultrasonic Lithotripsy of Large Staghorn Calculus. J.Urol., 131:1147, 1984.

13. Elyaderani, M.K., Belis, J.A., Kandzari, S.J.,Gabriele, O.F.: Facilitation of Difficult Percutaneous Ureteral Stent Insertion. J.Urol., 128:1173, 1982.

14. Finn, D.J., Palestrant, A.M., Dewolf, W.C.: Successful Percutaneous Managment of Renal Abscess. J.Urol., 127:425, 1982.

15. Fučkar, Ž., Sobol-Dimec,J., Dimec, D., Aničić, : Eight Years Experience in Echosonography of the Congenital Anomalies of the Kidney.Acta Chir. Iuy., 31:217,1984.

16. Kaye, K.W.: Renal Anatomy for Endourologic Stone Removal. J. Urol., 13o:647, 1983.

17. Krhen, I., Radej,M., Parazajder, J., Kovačić, M.: Percutaneous Interventions on Kidney. Proceedings of 8 th Congress of Yugoslavien Urologists. Split, 1984.

18. Lange, P.H., Reddy, P.K., Hulbert, J.C., Clayman, R.V.,Castaneda-Zuniga,W.R., Miller, R.P., Coleman,C.C., Amplatz D.: Percutaneous Removal of Caliceal and "Inaccessible" Stones: Instruments and Techniques. J.Urol., 132:439, 1984.

19. Lieberman, S.F., Keller, F.S., Barry, J.M., Roesch, J.: Percutaneous Antegrade Transluminal Ureteroplasty for Renal Allograft Ureteral Stenosis. J.Urol.,128:122, 1982,

2o. Man,D.W.K., Ransley, P.G.: Percutaneous Antegrade Pyelography in Children.Brit. J. Urol., 56:237, 1984.

21. Miller,R.P., Reinke,D.B., Clayman, R.V., Lange,P.H.: Reestablishment of a Nephrostomy Tract. Urol.Clin. N.A., 9:75, 1982.

22. Mitty, H., Gribetz, M.E.: The Status of Interventional Uroradiology. J.Urol., 127:2, 1982.

23. Mayer-Schwickrath, M., Ringert, R.H., Homann,W.:Perkutane Darstellung Ektoper Megaureteran.Urologe A., 23:35, 1984.

24. Narayan, P., Smith, A.D.: Percutaneous Nephrostomy as an Adjunct in the Management of Ureteral Calculi. Urol. Clin. N.A., 9:137, 1982.

25. Newhouse,J.M., Pfister, R.C., Hendren, W.H., Yoder, I.C.: Whitaker Test After Pyeloplasty:Establishment of Normal Ureteral Perfusion Pressures. J. Urol., 127:616, 1982.

26. OOsterlinck, W., De Sy, W.A.: A New Percutaneous Nephrostomy Set. J J. Urol., 129:466, 1983.

27. Riedmiller, H, Thueroff, J., Alken,P., Hohenfellner, R.: Doppler and B-Mode Ultrasound for Avascular Nephrotomy. J. Urol. 13o:224, 1983.

28. Sadlowski, R.W., Finney, R.P., Branch, W.T., Rosental, N.S., Sharpe, J.R.: New Technique for Percuteneous Nephrostomy Under Ultrasound Gvidance.J. Urol., III: 559, 1979.

29. Schmeller, N.T., Goettinger, H., Schullr, J.,Marx, F.J.: Perku tane Nephrostomie als primare Therapie der Harnleiter- Scheidenfistel. Urologe A., 22:1o8,1983.

3o. Schoenberg, H.W.: Percutaneous Stone Removal. J. Urol., 132: 543, 1984.

31. Smith, A.D., Fraley, E.E., Castaneda-Zuniga, W.R., Amplatz,K.: Percutaneous Circle Tube Nephroureterostomy. J.Urol. 127:29, 1982.

32. Watanabe,H., Watanabe, K., Shuno, K., Oinuma, S.: Micro-Explosion Cystolithotripsy. J.Urol., 129:23, 1983.

33. White,E.C., Smith, A.D.: Percutaneous Stone Extraction From 2oo Patients. J. Urol., 132:437, 1984.

34. Whitfield, H.N. : Percutaneous Nephrolithotomy. Brit.J. Urol., 55:6o9, 1983.

35. Wickham, J.E.A., Kellet, M.J.: Percutaneous Nephrolithotomy. J. Urol., 129:447, 1983.

Recent advances in ultrasound diagnosis 5. A. Kurjak, G. Kossoff, eds.

INTERVENTIONAL ULTRASOUND IN BREAST DISEASES

VELJKO VLAISAVLJEVIĆ

Department of Gynecology , General Hospital Maribor , Maribor , Yugoslavia

At the moment it is generally accepted that mammography is the only method with which it is possible to *detect* breast cancers with high accuracy. The most useful adjunct to x-ray mammography at this time is sonography. The initial optimism concerning the ability of sonography to detect early breast cancer has not been supported by objective clinical trials. But although mammography can screen nonpalpable , minimal breast cancer , it is not equally accurate in diagnosing carcinomas in all breast types. The tumors most often overlooked by mammography are those embedded in dysplastic tissue of high radiodensity that prevents radiographic visualization of the tumor. The efficacy of sonography lies in its capability to *diagnose* breast lesions. Because of the overlapping appearance of benign and malignant lesions , mammography should be used to detect lesions and not to decide about the nature of the lesion (malignant or benign). Contrary to that , sonography should not be used to detect cancers and to differentiate benign from malignant solid masses , because there is a significant overlapping in their appearances too , but the method is important as a diagnostic procedure in differentiating cystic from solid masses (1).

Interventional sonography advances a solution for some of these problems :

Cyst / solid differentiation by sonography can eliminate surgery in cases where it is clear that sonographic visualization of the cystic nature of mammographically detected nonpalpable masses caused some of them to be aspirated under sonographic guidance instead of undergoing biopsy.

A sonographic demonstration of the nonpalpable solid masses can in some cases be evaluated by sonographically guided aspiration of the specimen for histologic analysis.

Sonography can also be useful in a selected number of cases in permitting preoperative wire or needle placement for the surgical guidance and excision of clinically occult lesions.

Supported by National Research Foundation 09 - 3176 - 333 - 84 / 85

METHODS

All examinations were performed using Picker International 5000 real time equipment and 3.5 MHz biopsy probe , 5 MHz or 7.5 MHz probes. The patients were examined in the supine oblique position. The ipsilateral arm was placed behind the head , and the air mattress was laid under the thorax. The result of such a position was thin and relatively immobile breast.

The biopsy transducer was disinfected in a cetavlone solution. The skin was surgically cleansed using betadine iodine. Sterile paraffin was applied as a contact medium. Using such a technique we have not observed any complications (inflammation of the punctured site) for the last two years.

RESULTS

A. <u>Fluid aspiration and aspiration of cellular material for cytologic specimen</u>

After the skin is disinfected a fine needle is inserted into the lesion. Aspira - tion is accomplished by a Cameco[R] pistol for easier syringe manipulation. The disappearance of a cystic lesion during aspiration can be followed on the monitor (Fig. 1).

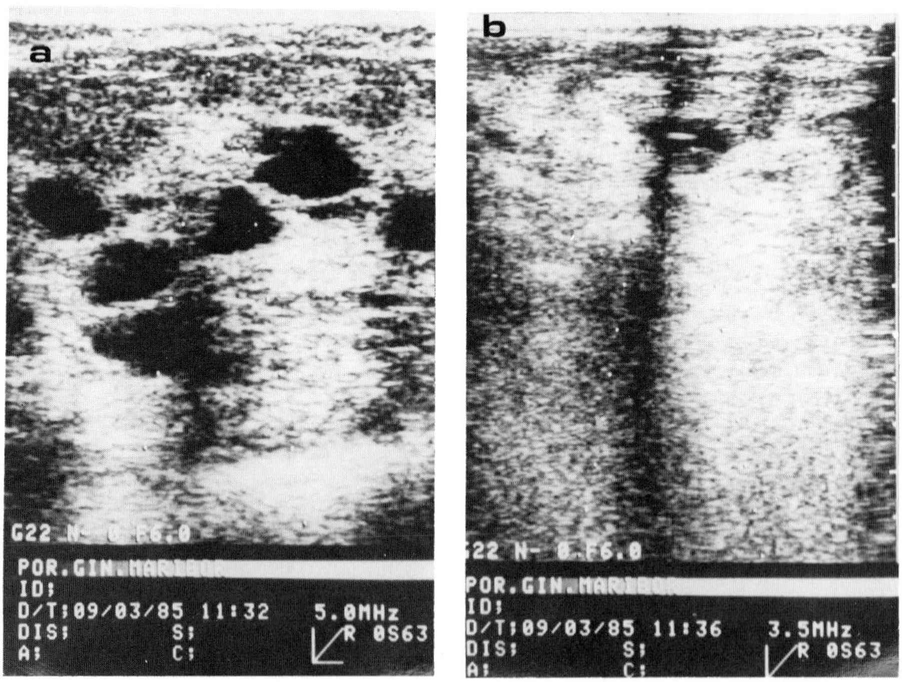

Fig. 1. Breast containing multiple cysts before (a) and after the sonographically guided aspiration. Note needle tip inside the cyst.

After the aspiration of the cellular material the needle is withdrawn from the breast and cleaned with a swab before the material is expressed onto the object plate. This prevents the mixing of cell material with drops of paraffin which could result in the disappearance of the cellular material from the object slide during the fixation.

The successfulness of sonographically guided biopsies of the last six months was investigated. The results are presented in Table 1.

TABLE I

THE RESULTS OF ASPIRATION BIOPSY GUIDED BY ULTRASOUND

Diagnosis	Aspirated volume (ml)	Punctured	Missed
	< 1	18	5
	1 - 1.9	29	3
Cysts	2 - 2.9	15	
	3 - 3.9	6	
	4 >	3	
Solid tumors		18	?
Total		89	8

In comparison to the success of aspirations guided by static sonographic equipment , which amounts to 70 % (2) , the success of biopsies under the control of real-time equipment is much greater , since it amounts to above 90 %.

Although sonography is superior in the diagnostics of cysts this is not of great importance in cases when the mass is palpable. The reason for that is the vital need for cytologic identification of all palpable tumors , and the act of aspiration will finally certify the cystic nature of the mass. A more important problem are nonpalpable cysts. These are small cysts detected by mammography but it is usually difficult to certify their cystic nature. The next problem is that the great number of breasts with cysts are radioopaque and the lesions are frequently not visible although they can be easily demonstrated on the echomammogram. In our previous paper (3) we reported on 35 % of such cysts detected by echomammography.

Before the introduction of interventional ultrasound such masses were classified only on the basis of their mammographic signs. This was risky because of the overlapping of the mammographic signs " typical " for the cystic or solid nature of a tumor. Unfortunately the cysts appeared in combination with benign solid tumors or cancers. In the group of 400 patients with gross breast cysts which were followed for five years, 17 times more breast cancers than expected and a 5 times higher risk for cancer during the five year follow up period were found. Benign solid tumors were found in 6 % of patients (4). These are the reasons why all breast cysts must be diagnosed and aspirated to ease mammographic interpretation. Such procedures dramatically increase the number of aspirated cysts in our Breast Diagnostic Unit. The introduction of echomammography in breast diagnostics in 1978 changed the frequency of cyst aspiration and pneumocystography. In the period between 1979 - 1984 there were 2.3 times more punctured cysts than in the period 1974 - 1978 (392 versus 921 cases) and less pneumocystographies (149 versus 64 cases).

B. Aspiration biopsy for histologic procedure

Needle aspiration biopsy is considered the first invasive diagnostic step in the diagnostic evaluation of breast masses. But unfortunately it is difficult to obtain adequate material for the cytologic diagnosis of all breast masses. The aspiration of adequate epithelial material from " normal " benign breast tissue in patients with benign breast diseases is often difficult to perform because of the predominance of fibrous tissue (30 - 40 %) and fat (50 - 70 %) in the breast (5). The aspiration of cancerous tissue which contains a relatively large amount of fibrous components can in a high percent result in nonadequate cytologic specimens. This is the reason for the need of histologic evaluation of sonographically demonstrable benign-like unpalpable solid lesions (Fig. 2).

The biopsy is performed by an Angiomed^{R} fine cut-biopsy-needle specially suited for histological biopsy procedures. The area of insertion is cleansed with an alcohol swab. One mililiter of 2 % lidocaini chloridum is injected intradermally and subcutaneously in the insertion site. Passing the skin and underlying breast tissue the needle is inserted over the lesion (Fig. 3 a). At that moment the stylet is removed from the needle and a vacuum produced in the cannula. The specimen is aspirated by turning and pushing the needle forward (Fig. 3 b). After the removal of the instrument the histologic specimen is pressed out and put under the usual fixing treatments.

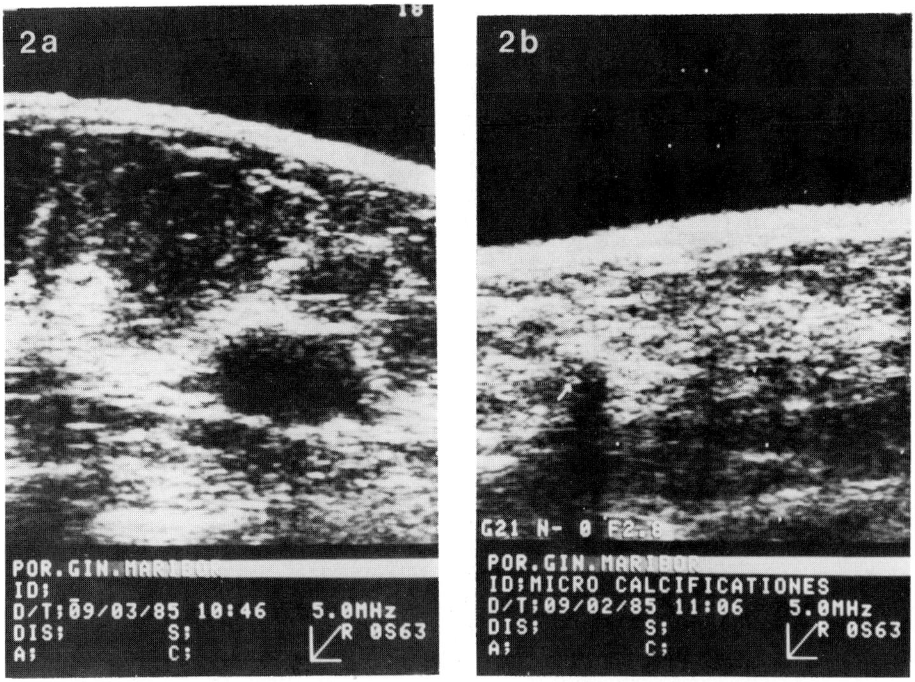

Fig. 2. Nonpalpable solid breast tumors detected by native mammography. Benign adenofibroma (2 a) and benign nature of tumor containing calcifications (2 b) were certified by sonographically guided aspiration.

C. Insertion of needles and wires

Breast lesions detected by mammography are frequently not evident in physical examinations. Many of them are not demonstrable by sonography and mammographic localization is the only method which can help the surgeon be sure that the lesion is contained in the biopsy specimen decreasing the time required for operation. For mammographically guided needle or wire insertion the lesion must be visible in the craniocaudad and mediolateral mammographic projection. In cases where the lesion is visible only on one mammographic projection the site of the puncture can be determined by sonography.

When the lesion is identified the needle is introduced through the skin close to the lesion. The needle is withdrawn and the wire or radioopaque teflon cannula is fastened with a strip of Micropore paper surgical tape. The tape is placed around the needle hub and across the skin surface. This keeps the needle in place until surgery. If the needle position is satisfactory in the repeated

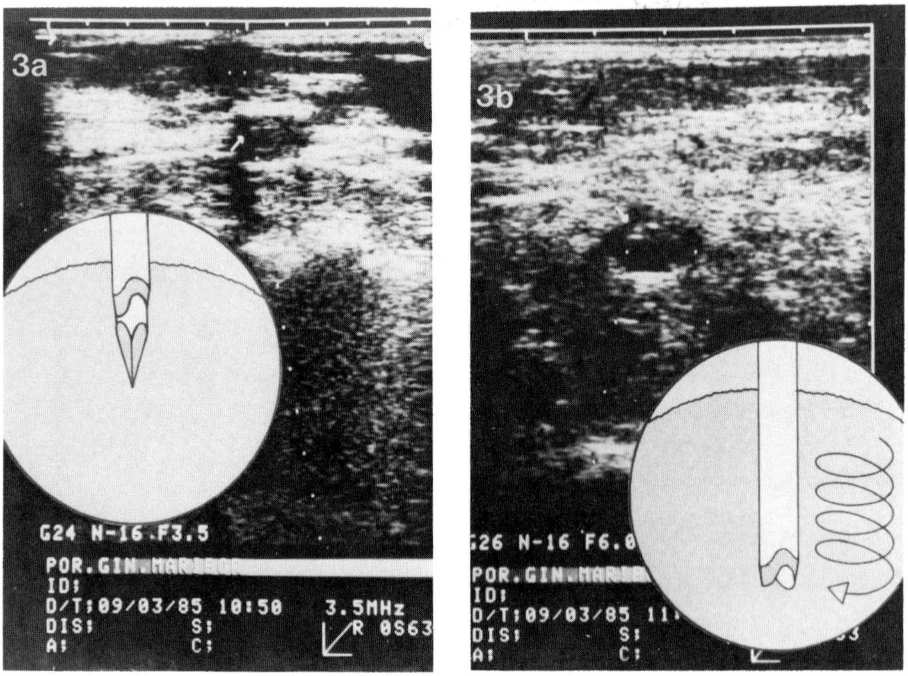

Fig. 3. Usage of the cut-biopsy-needle under ultrasound control. The histologic specimen certify metastasis of ovarian cancer in the breast.

mammography , a small amount of methylene blue dye is injected close to the mammographic lesion (Fig. 4).

Smaller lesions , which were not visible with the 3.5 MHz biopsy transducer , are localized by the 7.5 MHz linear array probe. When the site of the lesion is identified , the first needle is positioned under the probe over the skin. This produces the posterior shadowing which is a marker for needle insertion (Fig. 5). When the shadow is over the biopsy site , the first needle is fixed by the finger on the marked place. The biopsy needle is then quickly inserted through the skin and advanced into the breast perpendicularly to the skin in the calculated depth.

All inserted needles were certified by native mammography. Only in cases when the needle is not inserted in the appropriate place , the localization procedure is repeated on the basis of the mammographic measurements.

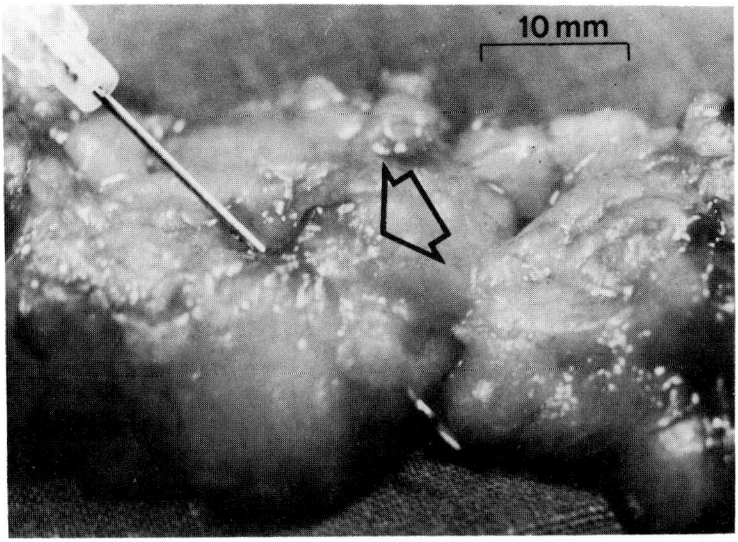

Fig. 4. Specimen of occult breast cancer detected by mammography and locali - zed by ultrasound. The site of the cancerous tissue (5 x 4 mm) is arrowed.

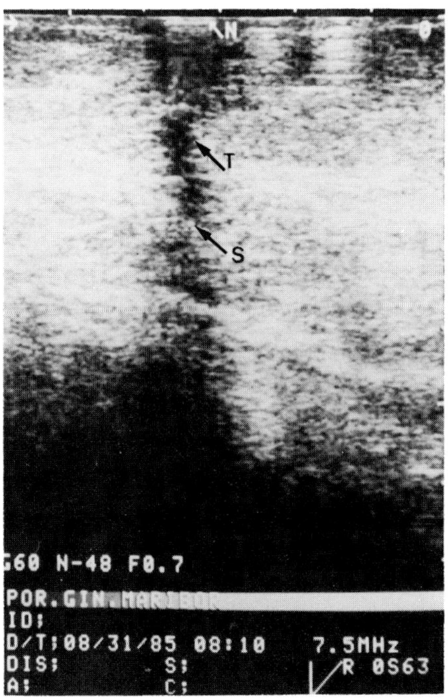

Fig. 5. The needle localization of the nonpalpable breast cancer. N - needle , T - tumor , S - acoustic shadow

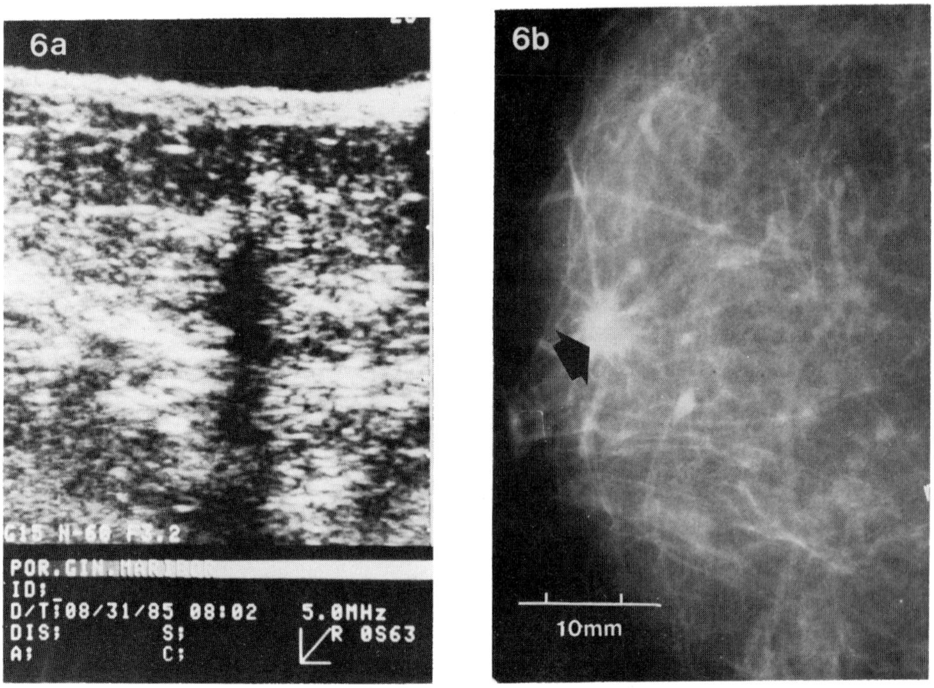

Fig. 6. Sonographic (6 a) and mammographic (6 b) appearance of nonpalpable tumor in 73-years-old asymptomatic woman. Infiltrating ductal carcinoma with the characteristics of a typical malignant stellate tumor was certified by biopsy.

CONCLUSION

We believe that sonography is most useful as an adjunct to native mammography in selected patients. A relatively new field for the use of real-time hand-held scanners is interventional sonography for the localization and aspiration of nonpalpable breast lesions. Sonographically guided puncture may prevent some unnecessary biopsies and eliminate all biopsies performed for lesions that are cysts. The method can be useful for the localization of many circumscribed lesions bigger than 5 mm. Unfortunately the method is relatively insensitive in patients with fatty breasts. The limitation of sonography as a method for the localization of nonpalpable breast lesions is in its inability to visualize most microcalcifications which are an important cause for open biopsy. The value of the method is still under investigation (6 , 7).

REFERENCES

1. Vlaisavljević V (1983) Receiver operating characteristic (ROC) analysis in determining criteria for the echographic diagnosis of breast tumors (Croat) Jugoslav ginek opstet 23 : 7 - 10

2. Vlaisavljević V (1984) Sonographically guided needle biopsy of breast lesions. Excerpta Medica ICS 640 : 49 - 52

3. Vlaisavljević V , Vrečer B , Gorišek B , Držečnik J (1982) Comparative study of breast tumor imaging by ultrasound and x-ray mammography. Radiol Iugosl 16 : 59 - 64

4. Vlaisavljević V (1985) The association between breast cysts , solid benign tumors and breast cancer , In press

5. Prechtel K (1970) Altersabhängiger Strukturwandel der weiblichen Brustdrüse (Flächenprozentbestimmung) Verh Dtsch Ges Pathol 54 : 393 - 397

6. Laing FC , Jeffrey RB , Minagi H (1984) Ultrasound localization of occult breast lesions. Radiology 151 : 795 - 796

7. Kopans DB , Meyer JE , Lindfors KK , Bucchianeri SS (1984) Breast sonography to guide cyst aspiration and wire localization of occult solid lesions. AJR 143 : 489 - 492

Recent advances in ultrasound diagnosis 5. A. Kurjak, G. Kossoff, eds.

ULTRASONICAL MARKING OF CATHETER

B. BREYER, IVO ČIKEŠ, B. FEREK-PETRIĆ

Medical Physics Department, University Gyn. Hospital, Petrova 13
Zagreb, Yugoslavia

INTRODUCTION

This paper describes physical and technological aspects of ultrasonically marked catheters; detailed clinical data will be subsequently published.

The use of ultrasonic echography in guidance of cardiac catheterisation could be perfected and find wider acceptance provided single plane imaging of flexibile catheters is improved. Ultrasonically marked catheters make positive echoscopic identification of the marked part possible (1,2,3). However, this method has some limitations that are to be discussed in this study.

Basically, the method consists of using cardiac catheters with built-in tubiform piezoelectric transducers (Fig. 1) which sense the incoming ultrasonic pulses when the marker transducer in within the scanning plane.

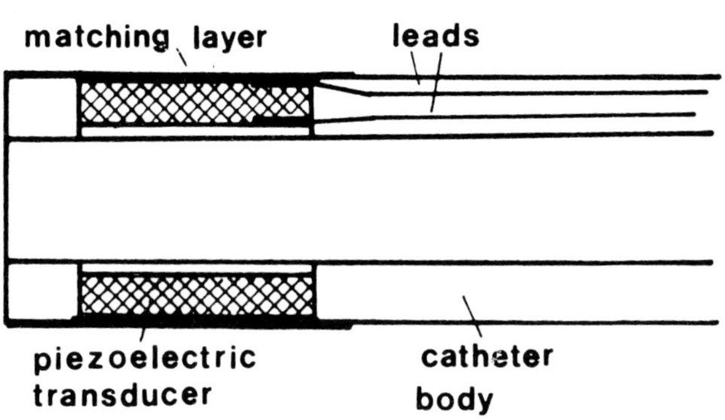

The electrical signal thus derived from the marker transducer can be used for generation of an appropriate mark within the ultrasonic image. This is done either using a passive system or a transponder.

The passive system measures the time elapsed between transmission of the echoscope ultrasound pulse and its detection by the marker transducer. This time is then doubled and after the double time, a signal is generated and added to the imaging signal. In this way, the round-trip time of the imaging ultrasonic pulses is compensated for and the marking signal put in correct location in the B mode image.

On the other hand, a transponder transmits a series of ultrasonic pulses upon being triggered by the echograph imaging ultrasound pulse, thus generating a mark adjacent to the marked part of the catheter (2).

TIMING ACCURACY REQUIREMENTS

In the transponder mode of operation the mark always appears adjacent to the catheter position. Timing limitation is the longest acceptable transponder reaction time. If a catheter diameter of 2,2 mm is taken as the minimal practical dimension, a mark that is nearer than 1 mm to the catheter image is acceptable. This means a reaction delay of less than o,6 μs, which is easily attainable.

In the passive mode of operation, the mark can be misplaced by appearing too early as well as too late. If the mark appears too early, the mark upper end will not indicate the catheter position well. Therefore one should consider the mark appearing at the top side of catheter image as the maximal allowable error which leads to a time doubling error of -1.5 μs, and if we accept the some delay error as in the transponder, a delay of + o,6 μs is an allowed maximum. In our passive system we use an analogue integrator circuit for time doubling. For these time measurements and errors of + 1.5 μs - o.6 μs at times between 15 and 300 μs, temperature compensation could be made even for absolute measurements. However, in our case when the times are compared within periods well below a second, no temperature compensation other than the use of modern integrated amplifiers and comparators is needed.

CATHETER DIRECTIVITY

The marker transducers are of cylindrical shape, sunk into the catheter body and covered with a matching layer, or membrane. Therefore, one would expect to have a nonisotropic sensitivity characteristics (4,5). The measured one-way sensitivity directivity characteristic is shown in Fig. 2.

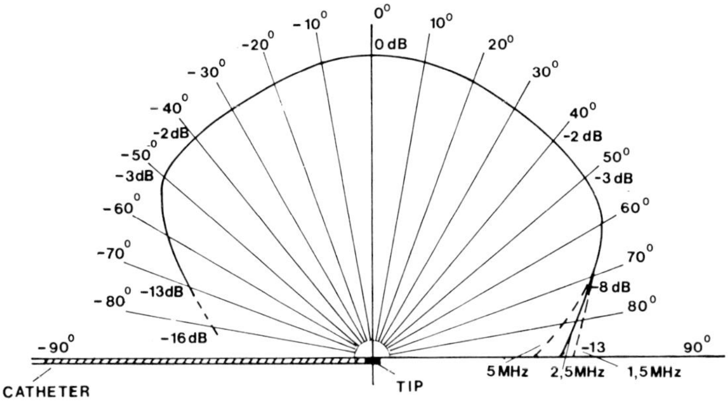

ULTRASONICALLY MARKED CATHETER DIRECTIVITY DIAGRAM
AT 1.5, 2.5 and 5 MHz PULSED ULTRASOUND

Directivity function of a tip marked catheter

Dimensions of marker transducers used during the experimental period are 2x3 mm to 2.7x3 mm. In all cases of practical importance i.e. scanning frequencies of 3-5 MHz the dimensions are larger than the wavelength. As a result the directivity characteristic does not differ greatly within the frequency range. However, one can see that there is a sensitivity dip of 12-15 dB at + 90° and virtually no practical sensitivity at - 90°. Thus, in order to properly use marker transducers, the dynamics of the scanner in use must have a surplus imaging dynamics larger than 15 dB, and the angles above - 80°. In modern scanners this dynamic requirement can be achieved practically. The influence of directivity is neverthless different for transponder and passive system.

In the transponder system, the directivity influences both transponder triggering as well as mark imaging at 90° incidence of scanner waves, the triggering signal will be 14 dB lower and the transmitted mark signal will be lower by the same amount, thus showing a fainter signal on the screen. In scanners with an actual display dynamics of 30 dB this can easily be accomodated especially since the mark is made to blink, thus having an additional identification difference.

Neverthless this must be taken into account in practical use since in pacemaker electrode positioning,using the four chamber view,such an incidence angle can normally occur. Another effect is resolution improvement, which will be dealt with subsequently.

In the passive system, the marker sensitivity influences only triggering. Once triggered, the displayed signal is always the same in amplitude. This signal, being electronic, and added directly to the ultrasound signal can be made not only to blink also, but black and white, i.e. opposite to the normal signal shade in the image. Actually, since the time and source of signal are known, the mark can be made to be any character via character generator, provided such an addition to the scanner design is deemed necessary.

INFLUENCE OF THE SCANNER PROPERTIES

Beam and pulse characteristic of the scanner influence the marker detection and resolution greatly (3,4,5).

Transponder and passive system are different in this respect. The transponder system is a roundtrip system, so that both transmission and receiving focusing influence lateral resolution while the scanner pulse length defines the triggerability time. As illustrated in figure 3 the sensitive volume of the scanner (space occupied by an ultrasonic pulse) differs with echo amplitude, while the shape depends on focusing, side lobes, and pulse length. In properly operating transponder on passive system it is the ultrasonic scanner pulse rise time rather than length which influences the response jitter. In order to avoid retriggering the response of the marking circuits must be blocked after the first triggering during the scanner pulse transmittion. A shorter scanner pulse has obvious advantages.

Lateral resolution in trasmission influences the triggering exactness in both systems. A narrower beam at transmission which can possibly be obtained by focusing and reduction of transmission power generates a smaller sensitive volume. In transponder mode it is the roundtrip sensitivity and focusing which influences both the scanner image and mark intensity. Therefore it is not possible to reduce the mark lateral dimensions below a level by scanner sensitivity or dynamics reduction. One can only try to use more extensively the better (transmit or receive) focusing.

In contrast, in the passive system one can act upon the mark lateral dimension partly independently adjusting the round-trip imaging sensitivity.

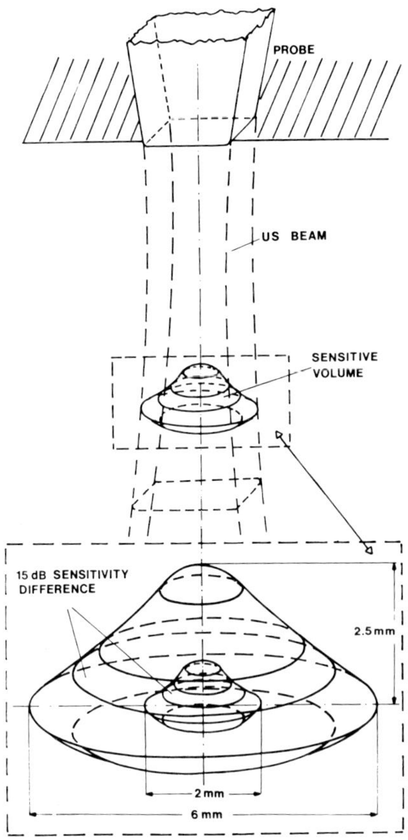

Illustration of reduction of effective space occupied by an ultrasonic scanner pulse when reducing effective imaging dynamics.

In this case only the transmission focussing influences the mark lateral dimension and one can obtain a narrower mark by reduction of transmitted intensity keeping at the same time imaging sensitivity at desired level by gain increase.

ROUTINE SCANNING PROCEDURE

The first task in routine scanning is to find the marker. In this phase a relatively poor resolution is of advantage for mark finding. The mark is easily identified by its blinking. Once found, the marker can be better localized with better resolution i.e. by using a lower triggering sensitivity and, for transponders, a better reception focusing. The sensitivity of the transponder or passive system can be varied with the built in amplifiers, so that it is not absolutely necessary to reduce the scanner transmitted ultrasound power.

Theoretically, but rarely in practice, retriggering by strong posterior echoes is possible, thus generating a spurious mark. Generally this spurious signal disappears as first at sensitivity reduction since an echo, appearing later in time, is normally smaller than the direct pulse impinging on the marker transducer.

In practice the catheter may, due to heart movement, move out of the scanning plane, so that the localisation signal is lost.

DISCUSSION

We discuss the applicability of these catheters as well as the associated electronics. Of the three electronic systems initially tested (2) only the transponder and the passive system proved practically applicable. The basic advantage of the transponder is its scanner independence, i.e. it can be used with any echoscope. Its basic disadvantage is the fact that the polarity of the mark is always the same as that of the imaging echoes. Isolation problems for the 5 volts used for mark transmission from the marker transducer can be easily solved.

The passive system advantage is the fact that its signal can be made of any polarity, even a character (a letter, triangle or other) is feasible as a mark. This is of special interest in multiple marking. The disadvantage is its scanner dependence, i.e. it is peculiar to the specific echoscope, thus the system can not be widely used until passive marking electronics is designed for the echoscopes in use. The core of the passive system (time doubler, modulator) is equal for all echoscopes, but the input and output circuits must be redesigned for each echoscope type.

The safety aspects must be dealt with in the way accepted for class C instruments, since the applied part (catheter or pacing electrode) is inserted into the heart. For transponders the easiest way to achieve safety is to use battery power and double isolated housing as is done in our prototype. For the passive system a battery powered input circuit and an optocoupler are satisfactory although one can use a DC-DC converter for power supply isolation. Unlike low frequency pacemaker circuits, the passive system is sensitive to frequencies usually used in DC-DC converters (0.9 MHz) so that heavy filtering is requierd.

The described technical problems have been solved to a degree that allows safe clinical trial.

REFERENCES

1. Holmer NG, Lindström K (1978) New methods in medical ultrasound, Report 1/1978, Lund Institute of Technology Code Lutedx/ (TEEM-1001)/1-420 pp 391-419

2. Breyer B, Čikeŝ I (1984) Ultrasonically marked catheter - a method for positive echographic catheter position identification, Med & Biol Eng & Comput, 22, pp 268-271

3. Breyer B (1977) In: Hinselmann M, Anliker M, Meudt R (eds)Ultraschall in der Medizin, Georg Thieme Verlag, pp 212-216

4. Čikeŝ I (1982) In: Hanarth P, Bleifeld W, Soquet J (eds) Cardiovascular diagnosis by ultrasound, developments in cardiovascular medicine 22, pp 178-201

5. Čikeŝ I, Breyer B, Ferek-Petrič B, Maliĉič I, Šesto M, Goldner V (1985) In: Dadd M, Gill RW (eds) Proceedings WFUMB'85, Pergamon Press, Sydney, pp 399

6. Breyer B, Čikeŝ I (1985) In: Dadd M, Gill RW (eds) Proceedings WFUMB'85, Pergamon Press, Sydney, pp 553

Recent advances in ultrasound diagnosis 5. A. Kurjak, G. Kossoff, eds.

REAL-TIME TWO-DIMENSIONAL BLOOD FLOW IMAGING USING ULTRASOUND DOPPLER

CHIHIRO KASAI, KOROKU NAMEKAWA
Aloka Co., Ltd., 6-22-1 Mure Mitaka, Tokyo 181, Japan

INTRODUCTION

Owing to the advancements in electronic scanning and high-speed mechanical scanning ultrasonic diagnostic equipment, real-time two-dimensional observation of the heart and other organs has been made possible.

In addition, considering blood flows in the heart and blood vessels, if the behavior of such flows could be displayed on a CRT (cathode ray tube) together with the tomographic images of the organs, significant contributions to diagnostics would be achieved. A real-time two-dimensional blood flow imaging system has been developed from such simple concept by our engineers.

For the blood flow imaging a signal processing technique known as autocorrelation is employed [1],[2],[3]. Explaining the technique requires mathematical analysis, but attempting it immediately from the beginning may confuse the fundamental issue. Therefore we will first make a qualitative description of the MTI (moving target indication) system often employed in radars, and then discuss the principle of the autocorrelation technique for better understanding.

In order to display blood flow images, we employ a color TV screen and the flows are displayed in color superimposed on tissue images which are expressed in monochrome. Later in the text the display process is described.

Finally, clinical evaluation of data collected in a hospital is presented.

PRINCIPLE OF MTI

In Fig. 1 when an airplane approaching an airport is captured by a radio wave radar, the screen displays not only echoes reflected by the airplane but also those by nearby buildings. If such buildings are numerous and their echoes are strong, the airplane echoes are buried within the building echoes and made difficult to identify. MTI is a technique to extract only echoes from moving targets like airplanes even in such circumstances. In the figure, the pulse waveforms shown below represent the echo waveforms obtained when two radio pulses are transmitted. Since the buildings are stationary, no radio wave pulse alters the echo waveforms. In contrast, the echoes reflected by the airplane exhibit a shift in waveform every time a radio pulse is transmitted due to its incessant dislocation, and when the plane is approaching the airport, its echo will arrive increasingly earlier.

Accordingly, by storing in some manner all the echoes obtained by a given radio pulse transmission, and by subtracting those from the echoes obtained by the next

* Illustrations 7-11 were originally submitted in colour, but had to be reproduced in black and white for technical reasons. Arrows have been added to indicate the colour definition as explained within the text.

pulse transmission, a zero output results for stationary objects. Whereas relative to moving objects, finite outputs are obtained. Therefore, when such differential outputs are amplified and then brightness-modulated on a CRT, only the echoes from moving objects like an airplane are displayed on the CRT. This is the operating principle of MTI.

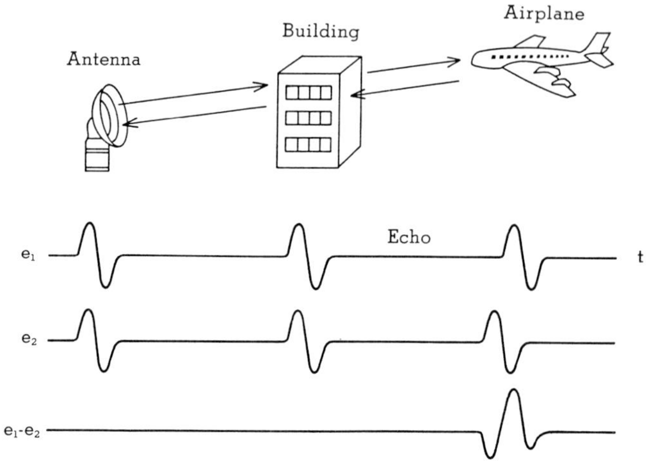

Fig. 1 Principle of an MTI radar.

Delay lines are often used for the temporary storage of echo signals. Figure 2 shows an echo signal subtractor employing a delay line. The delay time of the delay line is made equal to the interval of the pulse transmission.

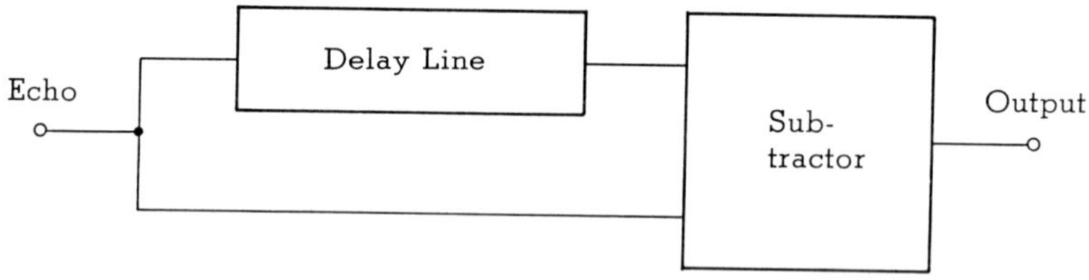

Fig. 2 Echo signal subtractor using a delay line.

Delay lines for the above application include not only analog types where signals are delayed in analog waveforms, but lately also digital types where signals are converted to digital data by the use of an AD converter, stored in memory and then called after a predesignated length of time.

In the MTI process, moving objects are displayed on a CRT screen as luminescent spots and the direction of the objects is identified by visually following the moving behavior of the spots.

BLOOD FLOW DETECTION USING AUTOCORRELATION

By applying the MTI principle discussed above to an ultrasonic diagnostic instrument where sound waves are used instead of radio waves, it should be possible to display blood flows in a heart or great vessels on a CRT. However in the case of blood flow imaging, the direct use of this technique makes it difficult to identify the flow direction.

This is firstly because of the large number of moving objects in the blood flow. If only a few moving objects were involved and their sizes were significantly larger than the wavelength, it would be possible to visually follow the movements of spots on the CRT. In the case of blood flow, however, the diameter of the corpuscles, which are believed to generate echoes, is far smaller than the wavelength, and the number of corpuscles is virtually countless. In addition, the corpuscles are spaced at distances much shorter than the wavelength. Accordingly, when blood echo signals are processed with the MTI instrument in Fig. 2, the existence of blood flow may be detected but its direction remains unidentified.

Thus, the autocorrelation method was developed to accurately determine the direction and the speed of blood flow. Figure 3 shows the operating principle.

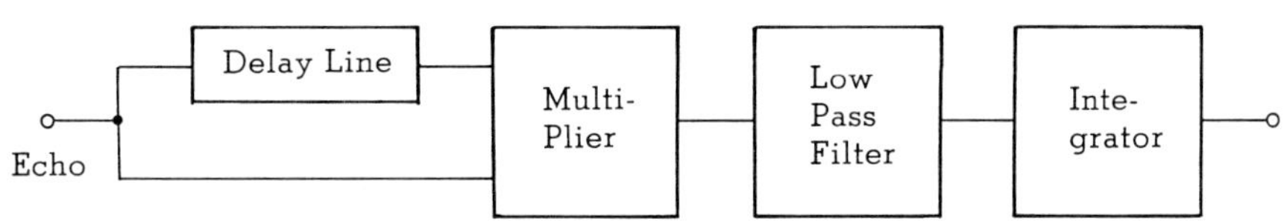

Fig. 3 Configuration of an autocorrelator.

Echo signals which have passed through a delay line are multiplied with direct echo signals of the next pulse transmission which have bypassed the delay line. The multiplier output contains both higher and lower frequency components as will be discussed later. Of these, the higher frequency components are rejected by a low pass filter, and only the lower frequency components which directly relate blood flow are extracted. These components are next supplied to a sweep integrator where their dispersions are averaged.

Now let us assume that a wave reflecting target is situated at distance ℓ_1 in front of a probe as shown in Fig. 4 and that the target is moving away from the

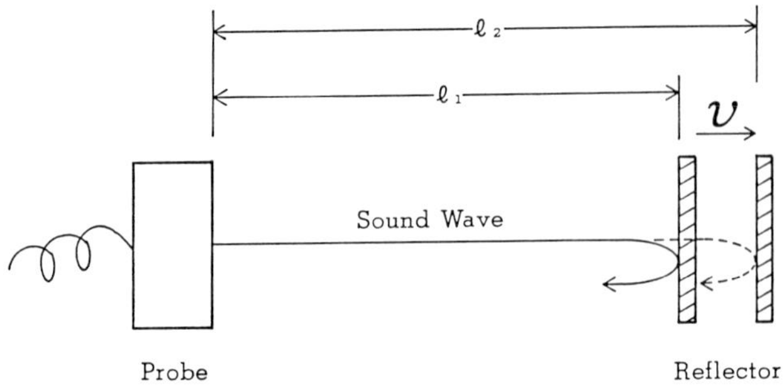

Fig. 4 Arrangement of a probe and a moving reflector.

probe at a speed v. By denoting the transmitting sound frequency by f_0, the transmitted wave is expressed mathematically by the equation below.

$$e_t(t) = A_t \cos(\omega_0 t) \tag{1}$$

where, $\omega_0 = 2\pi f_0$ is the angular frequency and A_t the amplitude of a transmitted wave. When the first sound pulse is radiated from the probe, the received signal reflected by the target may be expressed as follows:

$$e_1(t) = A_r \cos(\omega_0 t - \phi_1) \tag{2}$$

where ϕ_1 indicates the magnitude of the phase delay in the received signal behind the phase of the transmitted wave and it is expressed as

$$\phi_1 = 2\pi(2\ell_1/\lambda_0) \tag{3}$$

In Eq. (3), $2\ell_1$ is the round trip distance between the probe and the target, and λ_0 the acoustic wavelength. $2\ell_1/\lambda_0$ therefore is a quantity which indicates the number of wavelength by which the arrival of the received wave is delayed. A_r is the amplitude of the received wave and will be smaller than A_t, since sound waves are attenuated as they propagate.

Similarly, the sound waveform received by the second pulse transmission is expressed as

$$e_2(t) = A_r \cos(\omega_0 t - \phi_2) \tag{4}$$

where, $\phi_2 = 2\pi(2\ell_2/\lambda_0)$ and ℓ_2 is the distance between the probe and the target when the sound pulse hits the target.

Accordingly, it is easily understood that ℓ_2 is expressed as follows by denoting the interval of pulse transmission with T:

$$\ell_2 = \ell_1 + vT \tag{5}$$

In Fig. 3, by making the delay time of the delay line equal to T, the echo $e_1(t)$

which has passed through the delay line is multiplied with the direct echo $e_2(t)$ which has bypassed the delay line. The product becomes as follows:

$$e_3(t) = e_1(t) \cdot e_2(t)$$
$$= (A_r^2/2)\{\cos(2\omega_0 t - \phi_1 - \phi_2) + \cos(\phi_2 - \phi_1)\} \quad (6)$$

Ultrasound frequency f_0 employed in ultrasonic diagnostic equipment is usually at the range of 2 to 10 MHz, while the frequency of Doppler signal $(\phi_2 - \phi_1)$ is in the order of 20 kHz even with fast blood flow and it is far below f_0. For this reason, when the multiplier output $e_3(t)$ passes through a low pass filter, the first term in the large parenthesis in Eq. (6) is eliminated and only its second term emerges. This second term gives the Doppler component and it is rewritten as follows using the relative equations given before:

$$e_4(t) = (A^2{}_r/2) \cdot \cos(\phi_2 - \phi_1)$$
$$= (A^2{}_r/2) \cdot \cos(\omega_0 \cdot 2vT/c) \quad (7)$$

where, c is the speed of sound and it is related as $c = f_0\lambda_0$. $\omega_d = \omega_0 \cdot 2vT/c$ is the Doppler angular frequency and it is 2π times the Doppler frequency, or $\omega_d = 2\pi f_d$.

The velocity of sound which propagates through living tissues is in the vicinity of $c = 1500$ m/s, while the blood flow velocity such as in the case of mitral stenosis may only be at 8 to 10 m/s at the highest. It is therefore seen that Doppler frequency f_d is roughly on the order of two digits lower than the radiation sound frequency f_0. By measuring the phase difference $\Delta\phi = \phi_2 - \phi_1$ in the circuit of Fig. 3, blood flow velocity is calculated as

$$v = \Delta\phi \cdot c/2\omega_0 T \quad (8)$$

DISPLAY OF BLOOD FLOW

Using the autocorrelation technique, blood flow direction, flow velocity and the flow disturbance can be obtained. When the conventional B-mode echo data from tissues is additionally added, the number of information data which must be displayed on the CRT becomes four. To display these data, we have employed a color TV screen and displayed blood flow in color and tissue images in monochrome.

Figure 5 shows the relationship between the flow data and the color display. First, the blood flow direction was displayed by the difference in color. That is, the flow approaching the probe was displayed in red, while the flow moving away from it was displayed in blue. The flow velocity was displayed by the brightness of the colors and it was made proportionally brighter relative to the velocity. Next, the disturbance of the flow was expressed by the variation in tint, where the blending ratio of green was increased in proportion to the flow

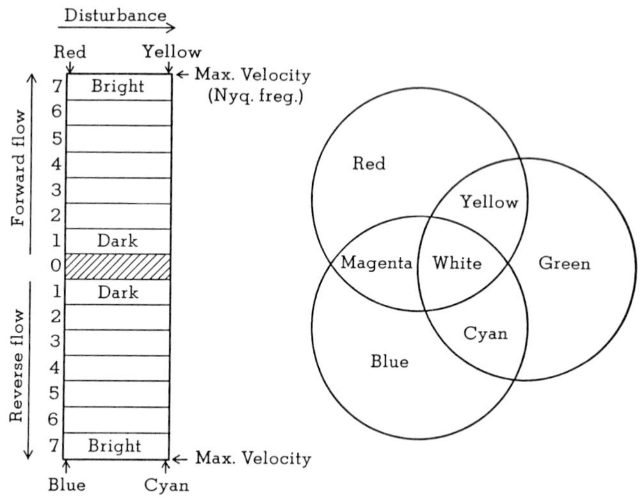

Fig. 5. Display of blood flow using color.

dispersion rate. Thus, the color of disturbed blood flow approaching the probe becomes yellow as a mixture of red and green, and that of flow moving away from the probe with disturbance becomes cyan, a mixture of blue and green.

Figure 6 shows a block diagram of this system. It is also equipped with the conventional spectrum analyzer to provide the spectrum at the sample volume specified.

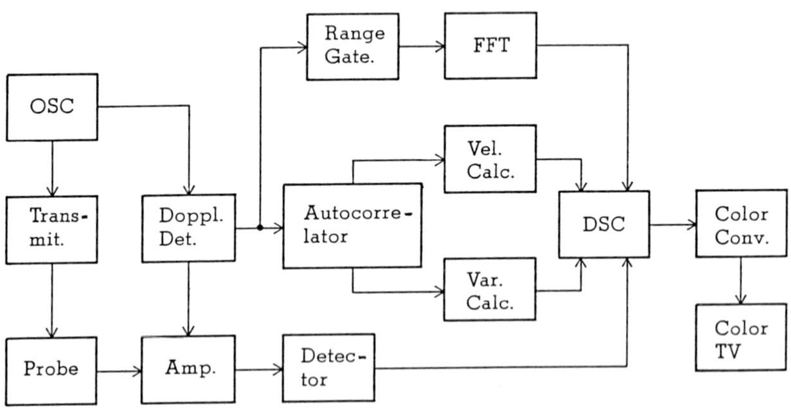

Fig. 6 Block diagram of real-time two-dimensional blood flow imaging system.

CLINICAL TESTS

Shown in this section are some of clinical data which have been obtained at a hospital using the system.

Figure 7 shows blood flow mapping in the heart of a healthy subject. The left is the image in diastole where the inflow from the left atrium to the ventricle is displayed in red. While the right shows the image in systole where the outflow from the left ventricle to the aorta is displayed in blue.

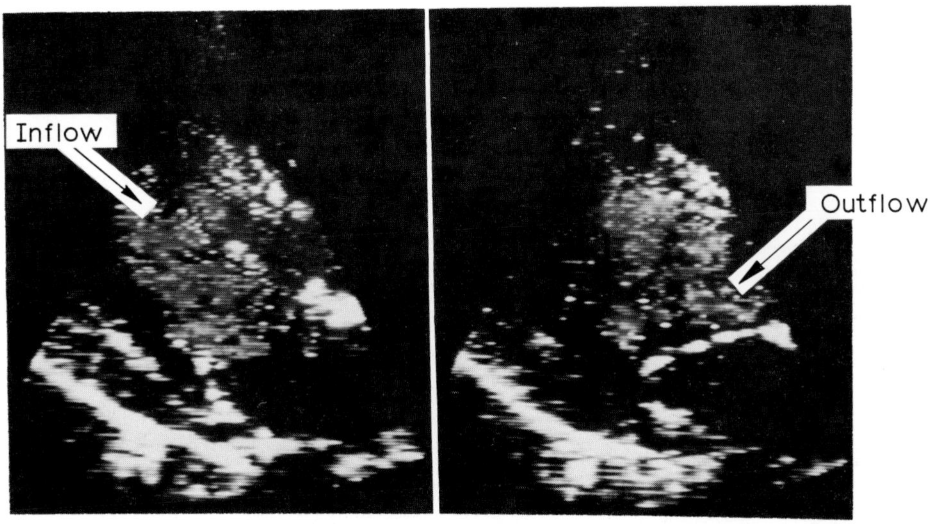

Fig. 7 Blood flow mapping of a normal subject.
Left : Diastolic inflow is shown in red.
Right: Systolic outflow is shown in blue.

Figure 8 shows the M-mode flow image in the mitral valve direction of the same subject. We can clearly see temporal flow variation accompanied by the opening and closing of the mitral valve.

Figure 9 shows the flow mapping of a patient suffering from mitral stenosis and regurgitation. The left is a diastolic image and it reveals a narrow jet spurt of inflow due to mitral stenosis. Since the speed of jet is high and the Doppler frequency exceeds the Nyquist frequency, the so-called color aliasing is seen where the color of forward flow is turned from red to blue. The right image is the one in systole, where besides the outflow from the left ventricle to the aorta, regurgitant flow from the ventricle to the atrium is also observed. By comparing the colors, it is seen that the regurgitant flow is more cyanic, suggesting that the regurgitation may be more disturbed.

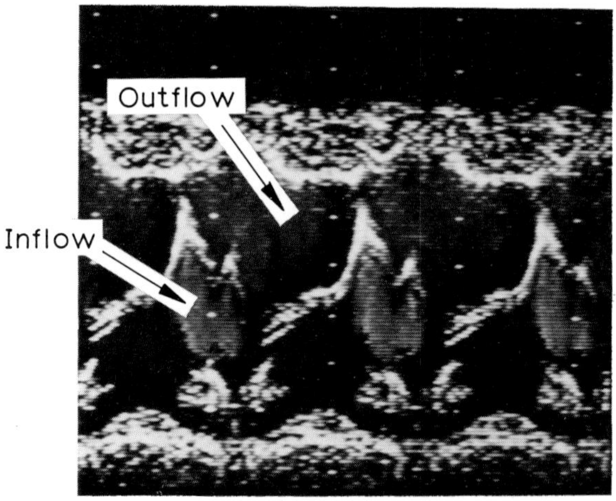

Fig. 8
M-mode flow mapping of a normal subject in the mitral valve direction in Fig. 7.

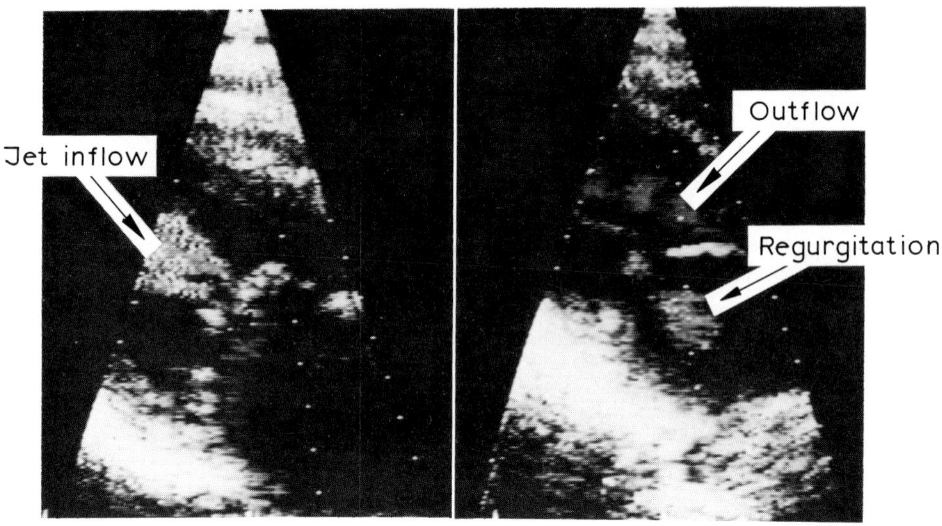

Fig. 9 Blood flow mapping of a patient having mitral stenosis and regurgitation. Left: Jet inflow in diastole is shown in red and aliased blue. Right: Regurgitation as well as outflow in systole are shown in blue.

Figure 10 shows the M-mode Doppler image of the same patient and it clearly reveals the relationship of the temporal behavior of the mitral valve and the regurgitation.

Figure 11 shows the systolic flow mapping of a patient suffering from tricuspid insufficiency, where regurgitant flow exhibits a mosaic pattern with reddish and bluish dots intermixed. This suggests that the speed of the regurgitation may be

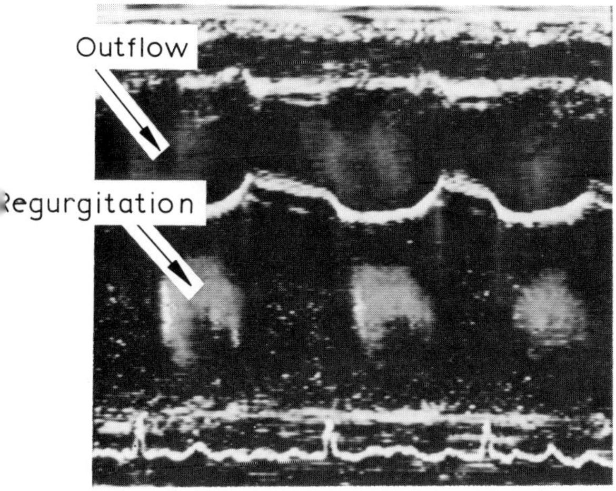

Fig. 10
M-mode mapping of the pasient of Fig. 9.
Regurgitation is shown as cyanic color.

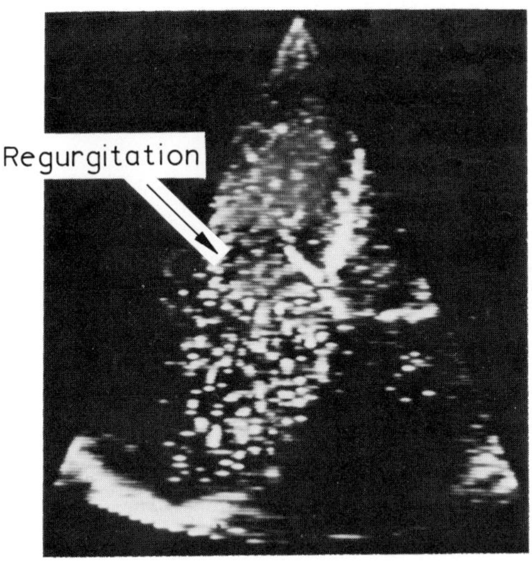

Fig. 11
Blood flow mapping of a patient having tricuspid regurgitation. Regurgitation is shown as a mosaic pattern.

very high and that the flow is highly disturbed. Though not shown here, when a spectrum was taken at any point in the regurgitation, it showed wide band patterns filled above and below the zero frequency line.

As presented in the above, color flow mapping not only detects the existence of stricture and regurgitation but also estimates the flow velocity and the extent of disturbance from the manifested color pattern. When a patient has a hole in the wall, shunt flow is observed.

CONCLUSION

In this article the principle and instrumentation of "real-time two-dimensional blood flow imaging" have been described, and the results of some clinical data obtained at a hospital have been presented.

At present, this equipment is mainly being used for observing flows in the heart and great vessels. But in near future it will be employed in the fields of the abdomen, gynecology, obstetrics and others.

ACKNOWLEDGEMENTS

The clinical data presented in this article have been taken at the first surgical division of Saitama Medical School. We express our sincere appreciation to Prof. Ryozo Omoto who kindly offered us the data.

REFERENCES

1. Namekawa K et al. (1982) Ultrason. in Medicine and Biology 8, Suppl. 1: 138
2. Namekawa K et al. (1982) In: Lerski R.A., Morley P. (eds) Proc. 3rd Conf. of Ultrason. in Medicine and Biology. Pergamon Press, New York, pp 203-208
3. Kasai C et al. (1985) IEEE Trans. SU-32: 458-464

Recent advances in ultrasound diagnosis 5. A. Kurjak, G. Kossoff, eds.

DOPPLER STUDIES OF THE NEONATAL CEREBRAL CIRCULATION

DRAYTON MR AND SKIDMORE R
Department of Paediatrics, Bristol Maternity Hospital & Department of Medical Physics, Bristol General Hospital, Bristol, U.K.

INTRODUCTION

The use of real-time ultrasound to identify cerebral haemorrhage and ischaemia in sick and preterm newborn infants is well established in many neonatal intensive care units. Despite this and despite the remarkable improvement in mortality of preterm infants over recent years, a few children are still surving with neurological handicap. Progress remains slow in reducing their number.

Evidence both from pathological studies after death and from ultrasound-scanning in life suggests that much of the handicap arises from circulatory imbalance which has lead to haemorrhage or ischaemia. Unfortunately ultrasound imaging reveals little of the circulatory conditions which lead to cerebral pathology. Doppler ultrasound may help fill this gap in our knowledge and so allow us to manage our patients in such a way as to minimise risk to the cerebral circulation.

Although several other techniques have been used to assess cerebral perfusion in the newborn infant, the major advantages to the neonatologist of Doppler ultrasound are similar to the advantages of ultrasound imaging. It is non-invasive, suitable for repeated use and therefore sequential studies and the equipment may be readily brought into the neonatal unit and used without disturbance to infant or his monitoring and life-support systems. On the debit side, Doppler ultrasound is not suitable for continuous monitoring and has very limited ability to assess regional perfusion within the brain. However the major problem associated with its use has been the difficulty in interpreting Doppler signals from the neonatal cerebral circulation. In the first part of this paper some of these problems will be discussed.

PULSATILITY INDEX AND THE NEONATAL CEREBRAL CIRCULATION

Studies of the neonatal cerebral circulation using Doppler ultrasound were first reported in 1979 by Henrietta Bada (1) who used a simple continuous wave Doppler system through the anterior fontanelle to record waveforms from the Anterior Cerebral Artery (ACA) (Fig1). As measurement of the vessel diameter and thus volume flow was clearly impossible, an indirect measure of blood-flow or vascular resistance was used, namely the modified Pourcelot Index of pulsatility (PI) i.e. the peak to trough excursion of the velocity waveform divided by the peak (Fig 2). This index had been shown in adult and animal peripheral vascular studies to increase as peripheral vascular resistance increased and blood flow decreased. It also had the advantage that it was independant of the ultrasound beam/vessel angle.

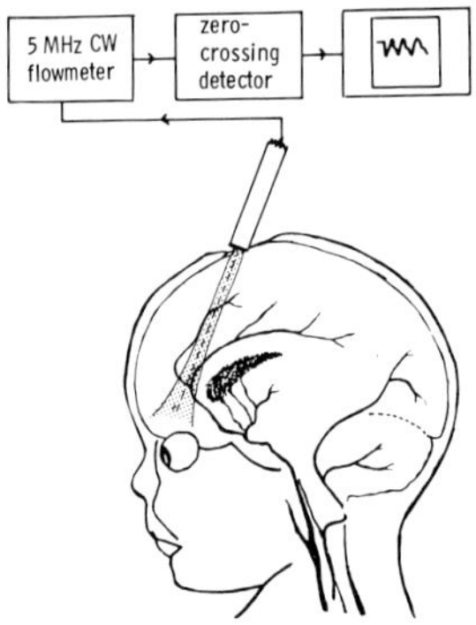

Fig 1 Simple CW/Zero-crossing detector Doppler system used by Bada.

Many subsequent investigators have used similar techniques but two separate attempts at validation of this application of the PI in neonatal animal models failed to show the postulated inverse relationship between PI and cerebral blood flow (2,3). Similarly in the human newborn, PI showed only a poor correlation with blood flow measured by the Xenon clearance technique (4).

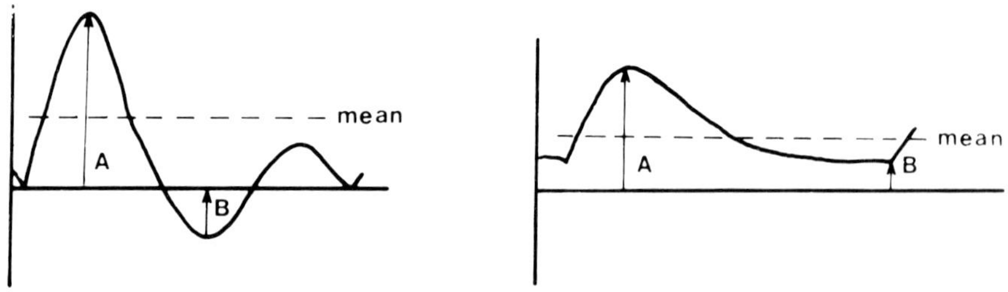

Fig 2 The modified Pourcelot pulsatility index (here PI) =(A-B)/A c.f. the widely used Pulsatility Index (here PuI) =(A-B)/mean

CARDIOVASCULAR EFFECTS ON THE CEREBRAL DOPPLER WAVEFORM

Because of the doubt over interpretation of PI in the ACA of the newborn infant it was decided to further investigate the relationship between the shape of the Doppler cerebral waveform in the human newborn and changes in cerebral blood flow. Short-term changes in paCO2 were measured. CO2 is a potent cerebral vasodilator and changes in its arterial concentration may be used to predict changes in cerebral blood flow. 20 pairs of Doppler recordings were made from the ACA of ventilated infants before and after changes had been made to their ventilation parameters, and arterial blood was sampled for measurement of paCO2 to match each recording. It was known that central cardiovascular changes (e.g. patency of the ductus arteriosus (5)) could also influence the shape of the cerebral Doppler waveform. Doppler recordings were therefore also made from the descending aorta whose waveform shape is likely to mirror the ´input´ waveform to the cerebral circulation and be minimally influenced by the peripheral vasculature. We quantified

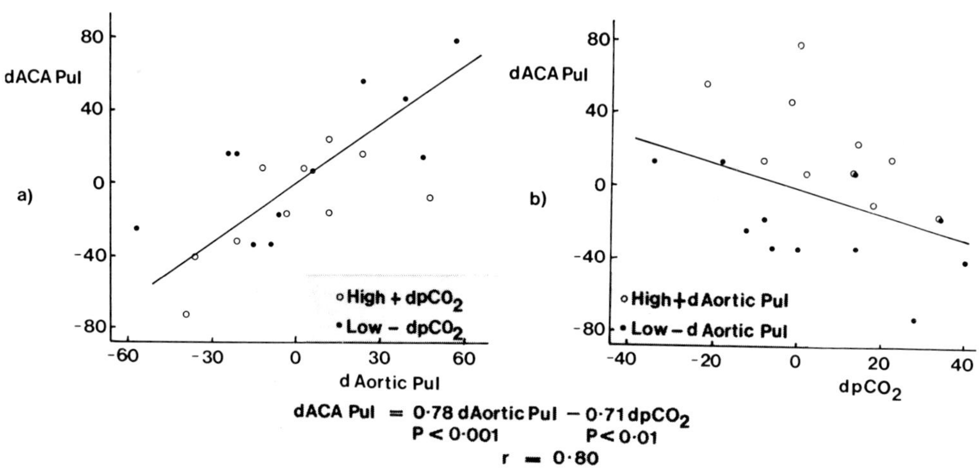

Fig 3a There is a positive relationship between change in Aortic pulsatility - ´the input signal´ - and ACA pulsatility change.

3b The inverse relationship between change in paCO2 - cerebral blood flow - and ACA pulsatility change is less tight. Central cardiovascular changes influence the cerebral waveform shape to a greater degree than peripheral vascular factors.

change in waveform shape using the fuller Pulsatility Index (PuI) - peak to trough excursion of the waveform divided by its mean (Fig 2).

From the regression plots (Figs 3a,b) it may be seen that although PuI does increase as paCO2 (and thus cerebral blood flow) decreases, the major influence on cerebral artery pulsatility is central cardiovascular change which is clearly considerable in these infants. The relationship is demonstrated more clearly in a three-dimensional graph (Fig 4). We have attempted to use this relationship by turning the regression around to predict change in cerebrovascular resistance or cerebral perfusion by measuring both aortic and ACA pulsatility. In other words if we know the aortic PuI we may calculate whether ACA PuI is higher or lower than predicted. Unfortunately the regression is less tight when used in this direction and results have been disappointing. However our conclusions must be that most of the reports of neonatal cerebral Doppler studies using indices of ACA pulsatility alone are not interpretable.

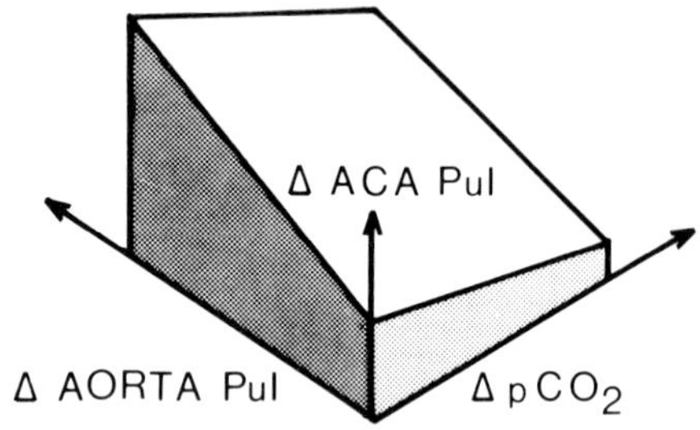

Fig 4 Relationship between ACA PuI, Aortic PuI and pCO2.

DOPPLER ANGLE DEPENDANT MEASURES OF CEREBRAL PERFUSION

Alternative approaches to the analysis of neonatal cerebral Doppler signals are to measure the maximum, minimum or time-averaged mean Doppler shifts (2,3,4). Two assumptions must be made if these measurements are to be considered to relate to cerebral perfusion.

1. As these measurements are dependant on the Doppler angle, the Doppler angle must remain the same between patients and between observations.

2. As blood flow is the product of mean blood velocity and vessel diameter, the vessel diameter must remain the same between observations and if groups of patients are compared they must have comparable vessel diameters.

The circumscribed ultrasound window provided by the anterior fontanelle of the newborn infant and the recurvant course of the ACA round the anterior portion of the corpus callosum allow one to assume that the Doppler angle is zero when the waveforms with the greatest Doppler shift have been found. This is made easier and more reliable if a Duplex scanning system is used which allows precise placement of the discrete Doppler sample volume with reference to the real-time image. A Duplex system may also allow one to achieve reproducible Doppler angles with other intracranial blood-vessels.

VASOMOTOR CONTROL OF THE CEREBRAL CIRCULATION

It has been widely assumed that there are no significant changes in diameter of the major cerebral arteries, growth apart. In most vascular beds vasomotor control resides in the precapillary arterioles. However recent evidence from studies performed on dogs (6) has shown that the cerebral circulation is unique in that even the large arteries at the base of the brain contribute 30% of total cerebrovascular resistance and that during vasoconstrictor responses to hypocapnoea or vasodilator responses to hypoxia or hypercapnoea, these large arteries may contribute as much as 47% of the change in total cerebrovascular resistance. They also participate in autoregulatory control and restrict the increase in small artery pressure following sudden hypertension. If these findings are applicable to the human neonatal cerebral circulation then the measured velocity of blood in cerebral vessels may not always be a good indicator of volume flow within that vessel. It would be easy to imagine circumstances in which for example ACA velocity was observed to increase while cerebral perfusion had either remained unchanged or even decreased.

A VOLUMETRIC DOPPLER APPROACH TO NEONATAL CEREBRAL PERFUSION

In view of these uncertainties of interpretation of neonatal cerebral Doppler signals, there has developed a healthy scepticism over the validity of neonatal cerebral Doppler studies. Clearly a new approach is required.

We have recently investigated the use of a volumetric approach to assessment of cerebral perfusion. In the neonate, blood flowing in the ascending aorta perfuses three major vascular territories (Fig. 5):

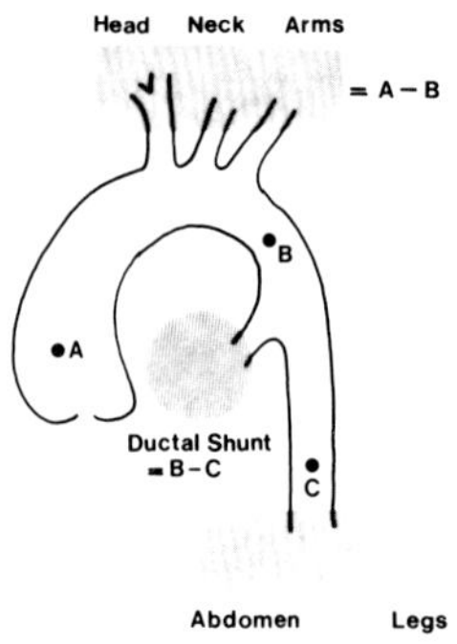

Fig 5 Blood flowing in the ascending aorta is distributed to 3 major territories.

a) head neck and arms
b) left to right shunt through a patent ductus arteriosus
c) abdomen and legs

Doppler techniques are now emerging which allow the measurement of volume flow along the course of the aorta with reasonable accuracy and thus the blood flowing to the three major vascular territories may be calculated by simple arithmetic subtraction. Our primary interest is in that proportion of blood flow which leaves the aorta before the ductus arteriosus. Measurement of blood flow in the major arteries in adults indicate that the great majority of this flow - possibly 80% - is distributed to the brain and so it is likely that this measurement will be a good estimate of cerebral perfusion.

METHOD

A Duplex mechanical sector scanner (ATL Mk600, Bellevue WA) is used (Fig 6). The blood vessel is identified on the real-time image which allows precise positioning of the range-gated Doppler sample volume and the direct measurement of the Doppler angle. The output of the Doppler flowmeter is the complete Fourier frequency spectrum of the Doppler signal. A segment of this digitally encoded spectrum representing about three seconds of blood flow is passed to an on-line microcomputer (Apple IIe). The signal in memory is then interactively thresholded to eliminate noise. The bidirectional maximum and mean frequency waveforms are derived and stored on disk together with Doppler calibration and angle measurements. The vessel diameter is measured from an M-mode recording and time-averaged velocity and indices of pulsatility and volume flow are calculated, the latter by using the average velocity/vessel area method. Two recordings are made at each vascular site and the results averaged to reduce errors in angle measurement and the effect of moment to moment biological variation in blood flow.

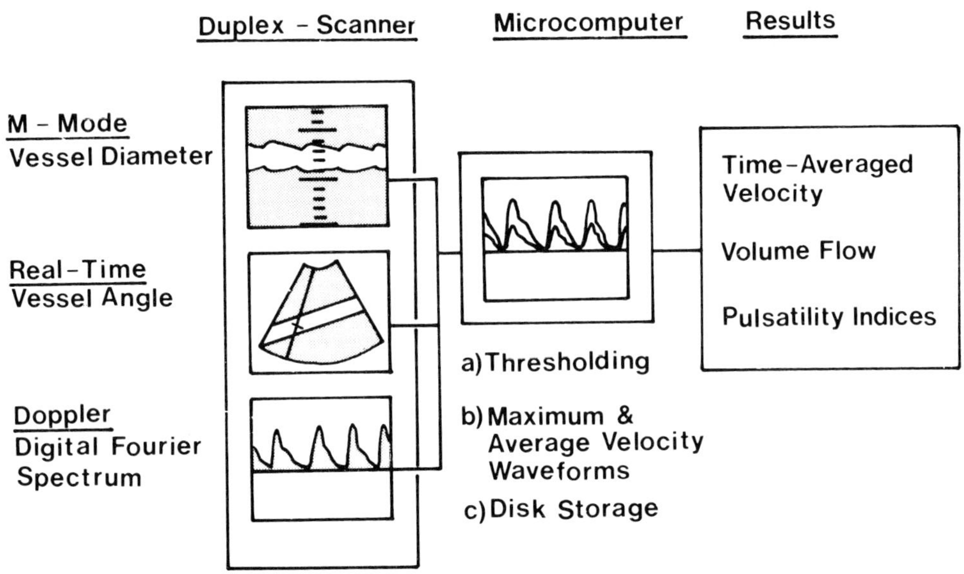

Fig 6 Duplex Scanner/Fourier Transform /Microcomputer system used in neonatal vascular studies.

The advantage of this method is that it provides an accurate estimate of the time-averaged velocity providing that the ultrasound is evenly spread across the diameter of the vessel. Other workers have used the maximum frequency envelope to calculate this average velocity on the assumption that the majority of blood is flowing at this maximum velocity (7) i.e. plug flow. This is not justified in the relatively small vessels of the preterm neonate (Fig 7) and is likely to lead to particularly large errors where flow is turbulent near a patent ductus arteriosus. Similarly the relatively simple analogue zero-crossing detector method of

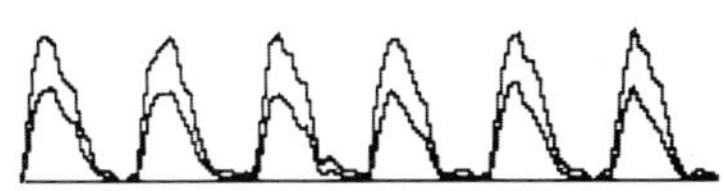

Fig 7 A comparison of digitally calculated maximum and mean velocity waveforms from the ascending aorta close to the aortic valve. The flow profile is ´plug´ only during the accelerative phase of systole, becoming more parabolic in later systole. The maximum velocity contour is not suitable for calculation of volume flow.

measuring average velocity is liable to large errors (6), particularly in the presence of turbulent flow. The achievement of an even distribution of ultrasound across the vessel diameter is easier in the small newborn infant than in the adult as it is easier to keep the sample volume large with respect to the vessel size.

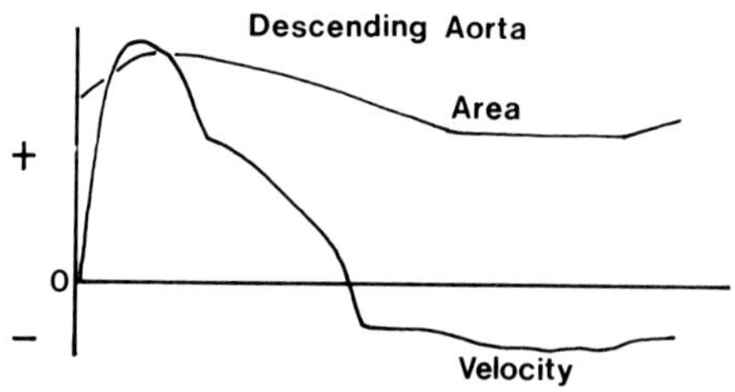

Fig 8 The cross-sectional area of the great vessels of the preterm infant vary greatly between systole and diastole. This tracing was taken from an infant with a patent ductus arteriosus.

Both the ascending and descending aorta in the preterm infant are very distensible. There is a variation in diameter between systole and diastole of more than 10% which may be demonstrated on M-mode scan (Fig 8). To calculate flow with ultimate accuracy it would be necessary to multiply the velocity at each moment through the cardiac cycle (V) by the equivalent vessel cross-sectional area. This is clearly impracticable in routine use. Our solution is an empirical one. The maximum systolic (S) and minimum diastolic (D) measurements of diameter are made. The cardiac cycle is split into systole and diastole based on the flow velocities. The instantaneous flows (F) during systole are calculated using Equation 1, and during diastole using Equation 2. Minimal errors were demonstrated in a range of newborn infants when comparing this method with the accurate one mentioned above and it is an improvement on methods using a single vessel diameter measurement.

$$\text{Equation 1.}\quad F = V \times pi \times (D + 0.8(S-D))^2/4$$
$$\text{Equation 2.}\quad F = V \times pi \times D^2/4$$

Doppler recordings of ascending aortic flow are made in the substernal 4-chamber view; of the post ductal descending aorta in a substernal long-axis view and from the immediate pre-ductal aorta in a suprasternal long-axis view (Fig 8a,b,c). Using these approaches we achieve Doppler angles between 30 degrees and 60 degrees. These oblique angles assist in ensuring even distribution of ultrasound across the vessel given the shape of the Doppler sample volume.

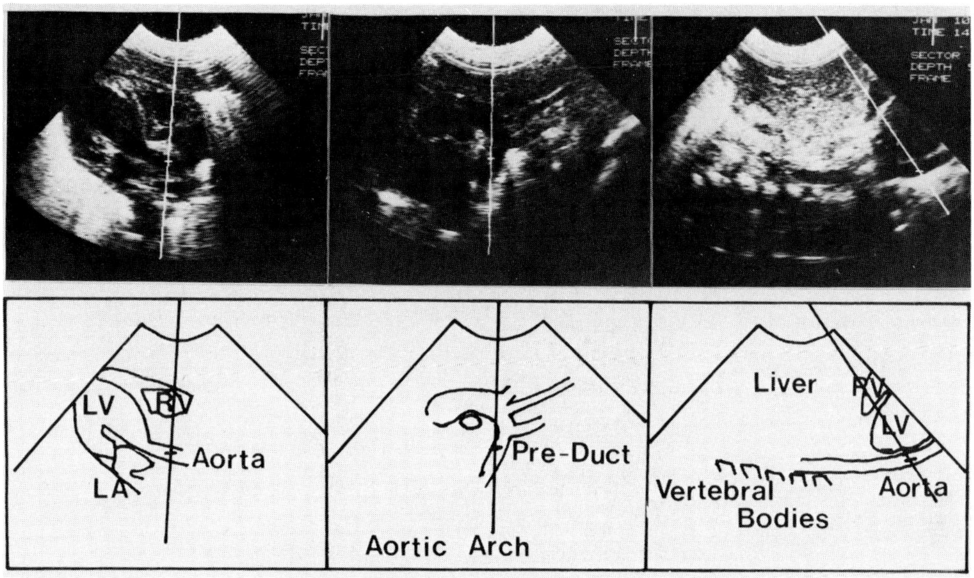

Fig 9 Approaches used when measuring Aortic flow in the newborn

a) Ascending Aorta close to the Aortic valve

b) Pre-Ductal Aorta

c) Post-Ductal Aorta

Intracranial Doppler signals are from the ACA in saggital plane through the anterior fontanelle and from the Middle Cerebral Artery in coronal plane scanning through the temporal bone.

PATIENTS

The preliminary results presented are part of an ongoing study and represent data from a consecutive group of 12 infants born at the Bristol Maternity Hospital of gestational age <=33weeks, calculated from the last menstrual period. Gestational age is confirmed by clinical neonatal assessment and in most cases also by early antenatal ultrasound scan (range 25 weeks 5 days-32 weeks 6 days, median 30 weeks; birthweights 940-2140g, median 1565g). Infants with major congenital malformation were excluded. Two further infants were excluded. In one the ductus arteriosus joined the aorta before the left subclavian artery making an appropriate pre-ductal aortic recording impossible. In the other, extreme irritability probably due to polycythaemia, prevented adequate Doppler signals and that study was aborted before completion. 6 of the 12 infants suffered from the respiratory distress syndrome. Informed consent was obtained from the parents.

Studies were performed sequentially shortly after birth and at 6hrs, 12hrs, 24hrs and 48hrs of age.

RESULTS

Real-Time Ultrasound - 10 out of the 12 infants had no abnormality demonstrable by ultrasound scan. One infant with severe respiratory distress syndrome developed an intraventricular haemorrhage and later post-haemorrhagic ventricular dilation. The other infant who was extremely preterm but did not have respiratory distress and received minimal respiratory support, had early signs of cerebral ischaemia with bilateral "flares" and now has cystic periventricular leukomalacia.

DOPPLER STUDIES - All results are median values for the study group of 12 infants unless stated otherwise.

Cardiac output and Ductal Shunt (Fig 10) - Overall there was little variation in cardiac output with time during this study, although those infants with larger left to right ductal shunts did have higher cardiac outputs (Fig 11). Median cardiac output at the 5 observation points after birth ranged from 181 to 213 ml/Kg/min.

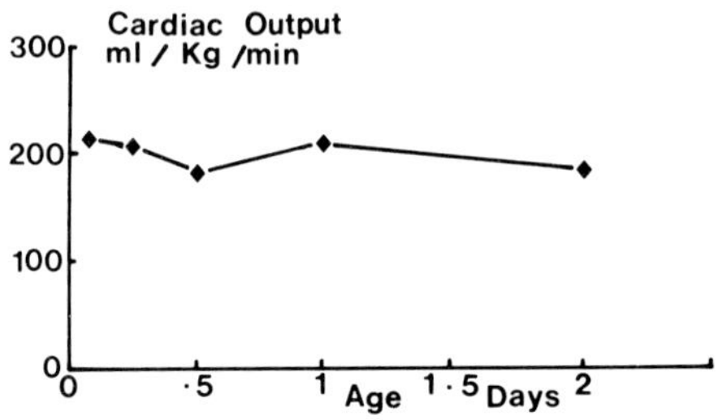

Fig 10 Cardiac output varies little in most infants within the first 48 hours of life

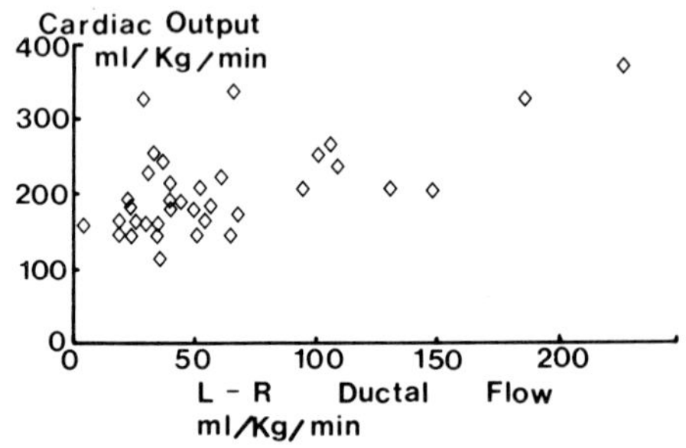

Fig 11 Pooled values from 12 to 48 hours. Cardiac output is higher in infants with large Ductal Shunts.

Predictably, the ductal shunt generally decreased over the first 48 hours of life (Fig 12) although in many infants there was an initial increase in the first 6 hours of life presumably as pulmonary vascular resistance decreased more rapidly than the ductus constricted. In two infants the ductal shunt increased progressively from birth (one subsequently required surgical closure). These two infants were the same infants who had abnormal cerebral ultrasound scans. However we were not able to demonstrate any significant decrease in "effective" cardiac output (i.e. cardiac output less ductal shunt) with larger ductal shunts (Fig 13). In other words the size of ductal shunt in these infants was not a major factor during the first 48 hours of life in determining systemic perfusion.

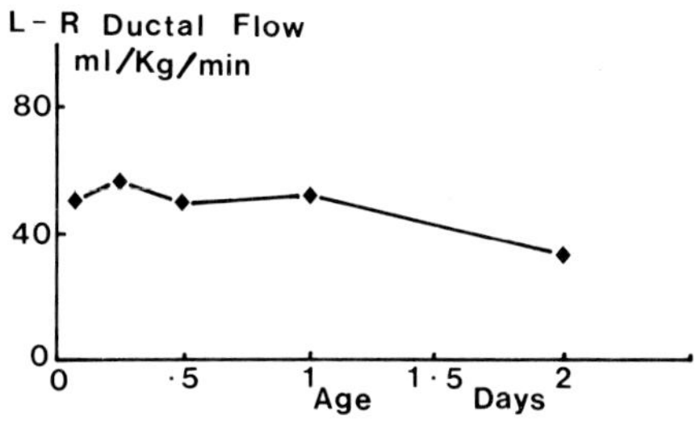

Fig 12 Most infants show an initial small increase in ductal flow followed by a slow decrease. Included in this graph are 2 infants in whom the ductal shunt steadily increased.

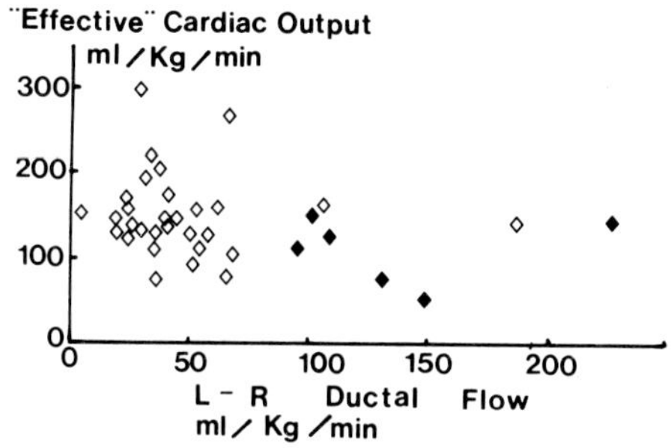

Fig 13 Pooled values from 12 to 48 hours. Cardiac output generally compensates well for increased ductal shunts. The filled diamonds represent 2 infants with cerebral pathology.

Flow to Head & Neck (Fig 14) - Between 43% and 49% of the cardiac output was distributed to pre-ductally supplied tissues. Blood flow appeared to be at its lowest at 6 and 12 hours of age, when it is known that the risk of periventricular haemorrhage is high. At 6 and 12 hours both infants with abnormal ultrasound scans had flows at the lower end of the range (Fig 15). In fact at both times one or the other of these infants had the lowest flow recorded.

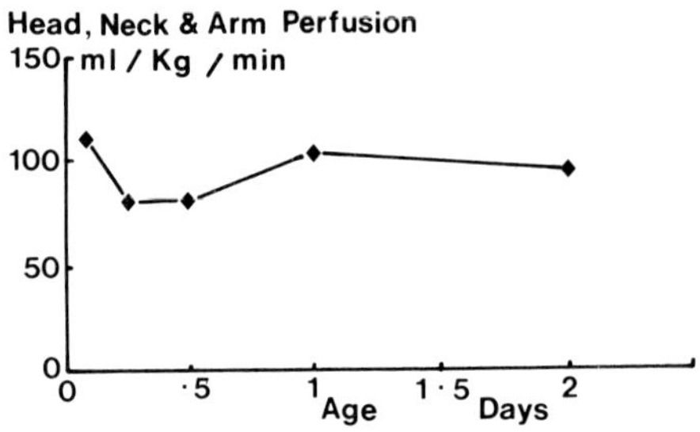

Fig 14 Lower flow to head and neck at 6-12 hours of age.

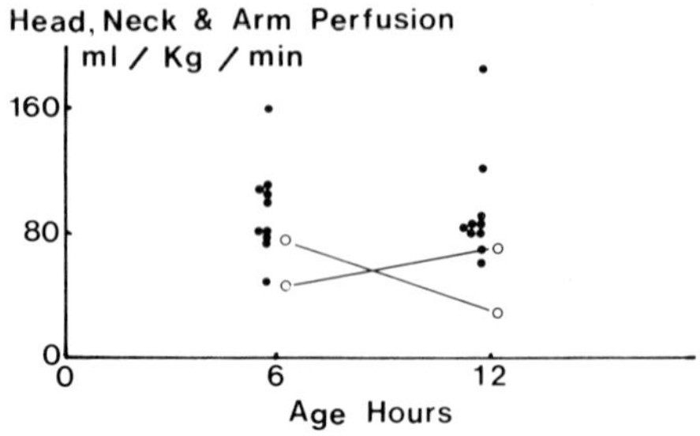

Fig 15 Distribution of flows to head and neck at 6 and 12 hours. The 2 infants with abnormal scans are represented by open circles - lines join observations from each infant.

<u>Intracranial Flow Velocities</u>

The changes in average flow velocities in the two intracranial arteries were quite similar to each other but showed a different pattern from the volume flow estimates above (Fig 16). Flow velocity was relatively low shortly after birth, increasing to 166% of the initial value (MCA) or 174% of the initial value (ACA) by 48 hours of age. There was no significant difference in flow velocities between the two infants with abnormal ultrasound scans and the remaining infants.

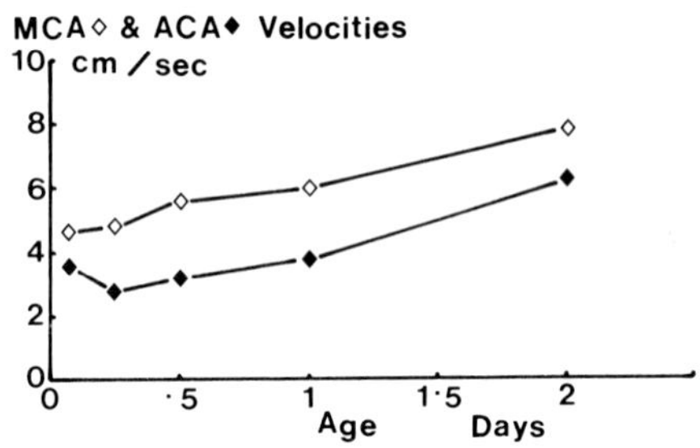

Fig 16 Anterior and Middle Cerebral artery velocities

DISCUSSION

Our measurements suggest that cardiac output is about 20% lower than reported elsewhere using Doppler methods in the newborn (10,11). The infants we have studied are not comparable either in post-natal or gestational age but we believe that the relatively simple methods of estimating mean velocity which have been used in the earlier studies may have introduced an overestimation of flow.

Volumetric Doppler methods are particularly susceptible to the introduction of error (13). In our technique likely sources of error are vessel angle and diameter measurement - errors which will be magnified when flow to particular vascular territories is calculated by subtraction. These errors are however randomly distributed (13) and may be minimised by making several recordings and by studying populations of infants. When we examine changes in flow over a short period (during which the aortic diameter may be assumed to have remained constant) one source of error is removed.

Although it has been known that in preterm infants ductal closure is slow and the ductal shunt is not usually accompanied by a cardiac murmur in the first few days of life (12), it has not previously been possible to make non-invasive measurements of the shunt to assess its haemodynamic significance. The majority of our infants were able to maintain adequate systemic perfusion despite moderate ductal shunts. However the two infants in whom there was progressively increasing ductal shunting both had low flows to head and neck and both developed cerebral pathology. Head and neck perfusion in the group as a whole seemed to be at its lowest between 6 and 12 hours of age. These observations have interest but it is too early to draw conclusions from such small numbers.

One of the most interesting observations we have so far made is that while the flow velocities in the intracranial arteries increase over the first 48 hours of life, the volume flow to head and neck does not increase in parallel. The middle and anterior cerebral arteries supply a large proportion of the brain and so velocities within these vessels are likely to be representative of the brain as a whole. If flow remains constant with velocity increasing then the vessel cross-sectional area must be <u>decreasing</u>. Indeed we may use the ratio of flow to velocity as a measure of the vessel cross-sectional area or degree of vasodilation. The difference between change in velocity and change in volume flow is then confirmation that in the human newborn, like the dog described by Abboud (6) there is vasoconstriction and vasodilation even at the level of the larger intracranial arteries. Plotting the flow/velocity ratio against time (Fig 17) we see that at birth the large cerebral arteries are relatively vasodilated, becoming more constricted perhaps as blood pressure and secondarily cerebral perfusion pressure rises.

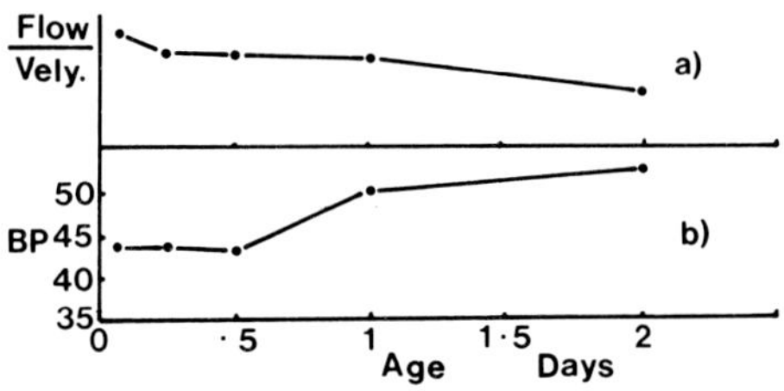

Fig 17 Flow/Velocity may be a measure of vasodilation in the larger cerebral arteries. Blood pressure is low shortly after birth and vasodilation may be necessary to maintain brain perfusion.

In this physiological model it is easy to see how during the early hours of life the dilated large arteries are unable to protect the delicate vessels of the germinal matrix from rapid short-term fluctuations in blood pressure so predisposing these infants to haemorrhage. At the same time if the large arteries are maximally vasodilated there may be no vasodilatory reserve to maintain cerebral perfusion should the perfusion pressure drop, and ischaemia might ensue.

Blood flow to the brain can only be considered with reference to the circulatory changes elsewhere in the body. When using a technique as complex as Doppler ultrasound it is also important to understand precisely what assumtions have to be made before conclusions can be drawn. In the neonatal cerebral circulation in particular, the pitfalls are many. It is unlikely that Doppler signals from the intracranial arteries alone will provide meaningful information about cerebral haemodynamics. The waveform shape is heavily influenced by circulatory changes extrinsic to the head, while average velocity measurements or ´area under the Doppler curve´ are influenced by calibre changes within the larger intracranial vessels themselves. However the careful use of Doppler ultrasound to measure volume flow is already expanding our knowledge of the complicated adaptation which takes place in the circulation of the newborn infant in the hours and days after birth. We hope that continuing studies will allow us to define more clearly the circulatory conditions which predispose to compromise of the cerebral circulation and the genesis of both haemorrhage and ischaemia.

REFERENCES

1. Bada HS et al. (1979) Noninvasive diagnosis of neonatal asphyxia and intraventricular haemorrhage by Doppler ultrasound. J Pediatr 95:775

2. Hansen NB et al. (1983) Validity of Doppler measurements of anterior cerebral artery blood flow velocity: Correlation with brain blood flow in piglets. Pediatrics 72:526

3. Batton DG et al. (1983) Regional cerebral blood flow, cerebral blood velocity, and pulsatility index in the newborn dog. Pediatr Res 17:908

4. Greisen et al. (1984) Cerebral blood flow: Comparison of Doppler ultrasound and Xenon clearance. J Pediatr 104:411

5. Perlman JM et al. (1981) The effect of patent ductus arteriosus on flow velocity in the anterior cerebral arteries: Ductal steal in the premature newborn infant. J Pediatr 99:767

6. Abboud FM (1981) Special characteristics of the cerebral circulation. Fed Proc 40:2296

7. Skjaerpe T et al. (1985) In: Hatle L, Angelsen B (eds) Doppler ultrasound in cardiology. Lea & Febiger, Philadelphia pp 306-320

8. Alverson DC et al (1982) Noninvasive pulsed Doppler determination of cardiac output in neonates and children. J Pediatr 101:46

9. Lunt MJ (1975) Accuracy and limitations of the ultrasonic Doppler blood velocimeter and zero-crossing detector. Ultrasound in Med & Biol 2:1

10. Walther FJ et al (1985) Cardiac output in infants of insulin-dependent diabetic mothers. J Pediatr 107:109

11. Alverson et al (1983) Effect of patent ductus arteriosus on left ventricular output in premature infants. J Pediatr 102:754

12. McGrath et al (1978) The silent ductus arteriosus. J Pediatr 93:110

13. Gill RW (1985) Measurement of blood flow by ultrasound: Accuracy and sources of error. Ultrasound in Med & Biol 11:625

Recent advances in ultrasound diagnosis 5. A. Kurjak, G. Kossoff, eds.

NEW ULTRASONIC TECHNIQUE FOR ASSESSING CIRCULATION IN FEMALE PELVIS

ASIM KURJAK and DAVOR JURKOVIĆ
Ultrasonic Institute, University of Zagreb, General hospital "Dr Josip Kajfeš", Pavleka Miškine 64, Zagreb, Yugoslavia

INTRODUCTION

The analysis of the Doppler ultrasound waveform is now widely accepted as a means of studying peripherial arterial occlusive disease (1). The continuous wave is commonly used for this purpose.

In obstetrics this method was introduced in 1977 by Fitzgerald and Drumm (2), who recorded signals from the umbilical cord. In the moving fetus the vessels are deep lying and their position in relation to the ultrasound beam is unknown making it difficult to keep them in the path of the beam.
The pulsed wave Doppler which is depth selective permits the assessment of deep lying vessels, the fetal umbilical vein and the fetal aorta (3). Depth selection is achieved by imposing a time delay in the reception of echoes from the transmited pulse. The position and the volume of the sample along the beam axis determinates a time delay as well as the length of reception time. The sample position is controlled on the B-scan which can be used aletrnately with the Doppler system. Using the pulsed Doppler and the B-scan imaging, Gill has developed the technique of blood flow volume estimation in deep lying vessels (4).

If a real time scanner is combined with a pulsed Doppler system it is possible to perform the B-scan imaging and the Doppler insonation simultaneously. Eik-Nes et al. were the first who introduced such a system in obstetrics (5). Using a similar system (6), Campbell et al. have recently developed a new technique for assessment of uteroplacental blood flow (7).

Based on Kratochwil's first ovarian demonstrations by ultrasound (8), this method is accepted for visualization of organs and vascular structures in the female pelvis. Thin vessels such as the ovarian artery and vein can clearly be identified as being always close to the ovaries (9). Despite this fact a technique of blood flow measurement in these vessels has yet not been described (10).

In this study, we have examined velocity waveforms recorded in the female pelvis from the vessels which had been previously visualized using the standard real-time imaging system, and have established a typical echo pattern for each vessel.

SUBJECTS AND METHODS

A 3,5 MHz real-time sector scanner (Aloka SSD 280) was first used for the visualization of anatomical structures within the pelvis. The full bladder technique was the basic prerequisite in obtaining a good image. Transversal, longitudinal and oblique scans were performed to identify the exact position of the uterus and the ovaries. Iliac, ovarian and uterine vessels and their position regarding the uterus and the ovaries were identified. Schemes of anatomical relations and vessel diameters were made for each woman.

A 3,5 MHz real-time linear array scanner combined with a 2 MHz pulsed Doppler, offset at a fixed angle of 52° (Kranzbüchler 8130 pulsed Doppler duplex), was used for assessing the flow velocity waveforms. The linear array imaging system does not provide as good an image as the sector system, but the uterus and the ovaries can be clearly identified. The sample was placed on the previously defined points in order to obtain signals or directly over the vessel which was possible to visualize. The Doppler signals were processed and displayed by way of an on-line spectrum analyser. The probe position was adjusted to give the clearest and the most representative signals free from artifacts. The records were stored on a magnetic tape for further analysis. The sample volume varied from 4 to 11 mm depending on the diameter of the insonated vessel. After examining one side the probe was rotated to take adventage of the propagation of the Doppler beam through a fluid filled bladder.

Blood flow velocity waveforms were obtained from 4 healthy volunteers (age 18-19) and 25 infertile patients (age 26-32) who attended the infertility clinic for various reasons. In all the women involved in the study a daily monitoring of follicular growth was simultaneously performed. The waveform analysis was made only in a situations where a normal follicular growth pattern was recognized (11).

RESULTS

Velocity waveforms were obtained from external and internal iliac arteries in 96,5% (56/58) and 92% (52/58) of cases respectively. These vessels can regularly be visualized by the sector scan. The external iliac artery is seen as an angulating transducer towards the lateral pelvic wall and the linear scanner, due to the great diameter of the vessel, is sufficient for visualization. The external iliac artery waveform is almost the same as the waveforms obtained from the femoral arteries consisting of a primary wave in systole followed by a reverse flow and tertiary waves in diastole (Fig. 1 AB). The internal iliac artery is usually visualized by performing an oblique lateral scan posterior to the ovaries. The waveforms from the internal iliac showed lower pulsatility, marking a diastolic flow and turbulent effects (Fig. 2 AB).

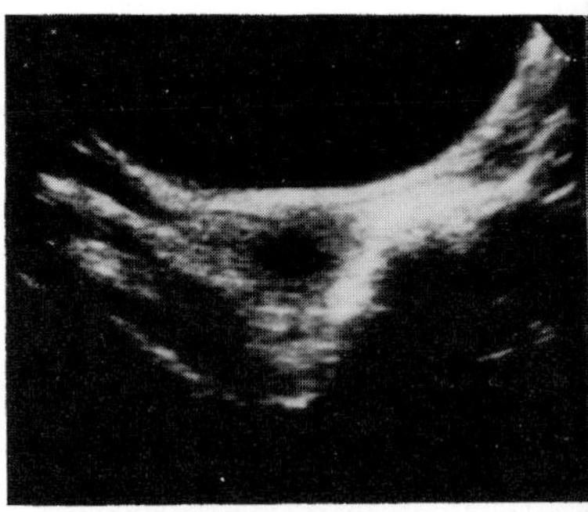

Fig. 1 A

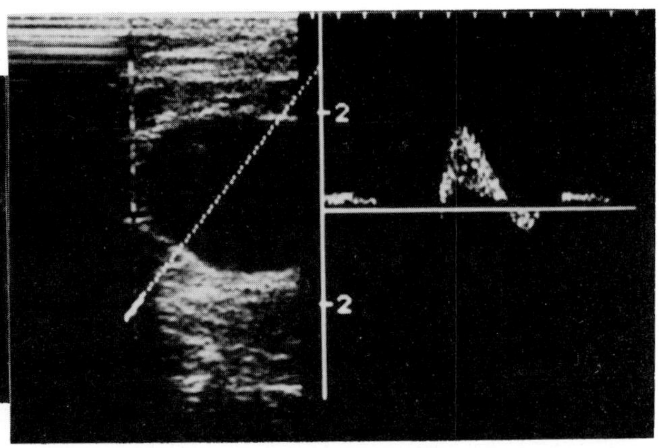

Fig. 1 B

Fig. 1 A - External iliac artery on the right pelvic wall.

Fig. 1 B - B-mode scan through the pelvis with marked sample position (left) and typical external artery waveform (right).

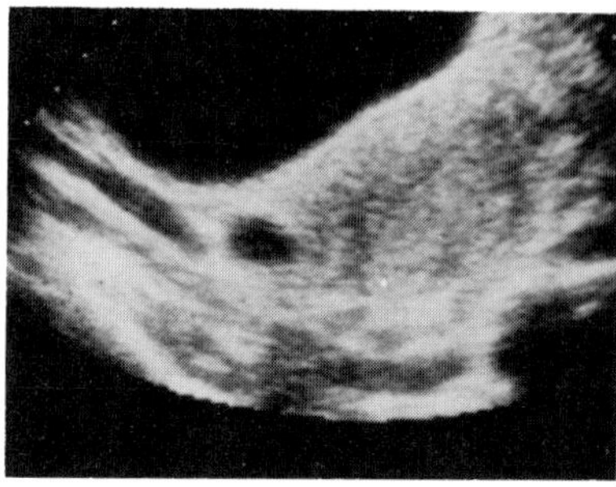

Fig. 2 A

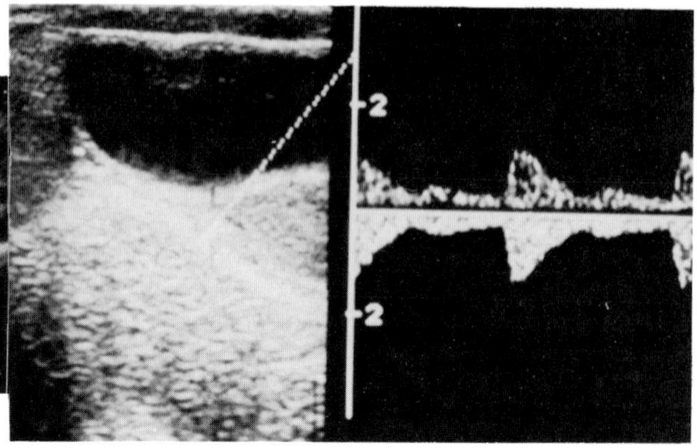

Fig. 2 B

Fig. 2 A - Internal iliac artery passing posterior and lateral to the right ovary.

Fig. 2 B - The sample is placed over internal iliac artery (left) and waveform showing turbulence and sustained diastolic flow is recognized (right).

Ovarian arteries were seen in 65,5% (38/58) of cases (Fig. 3 A). Doppler signals were recorded in 71% (27/38). Placing the sample

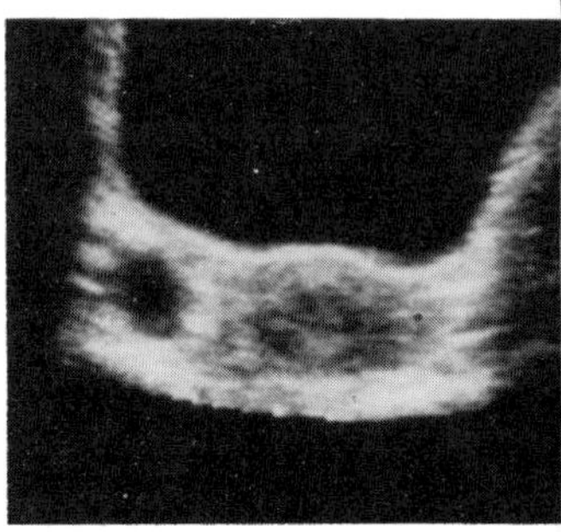

Fig. 3 A

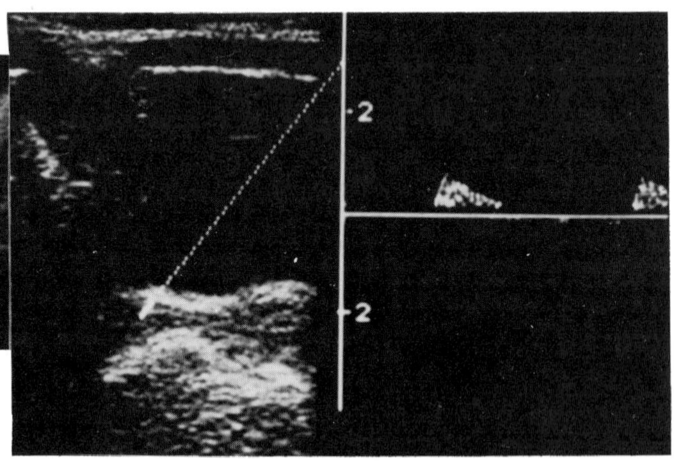

Fig. 3 B

on the anterior and lateral ovarian parts we obtained signals believed to represent the ovarian flow in 55% (11/20) non-visualized ovarian arteries. The inability to visualize the ovarian vessels occured in the case of lateral and high ovaries, when the lateral parts were covered with intestinal loops. Two types of waveforms were recognized from the ovarian arteries: low amplitude with no diastolic flow and higher amplitude with a poor diastolic flow (Fig. 3 B,C).

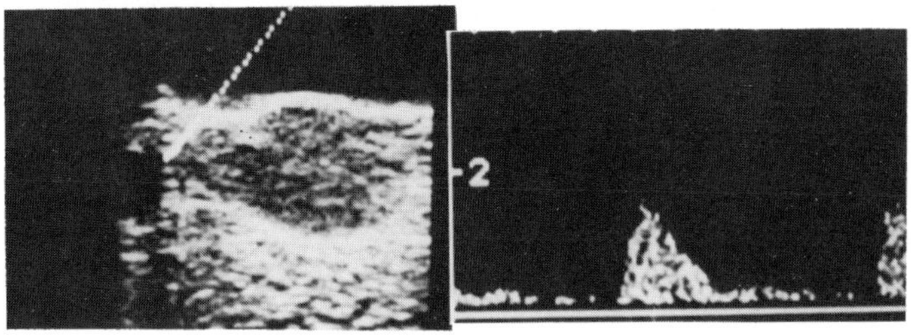

Fig. 3 C

Fig. 3 A - Ovarian vessels reaching the right ovary. The mature follicle is also visualized.

Fig. 3 B - The sample is placed on the lateral and anterior part of the left ovary (left) and low amplitude signal with no diastolic flow is recorded (right).

Fig. 3 C - Higher amplitude signal with small diastolic flow (right) is recorded from the previously visualized left ovarian artery.

In 9 cases it was possible to see thin vessels originating at the lateral upper part of the uterus and reaching the medial anterior ovarian surface, believed to be the ovarian ramus of the uterine artery (Fig. 4 A). The velocity waveform obtained from this vessels was very similar to the ovarian one, showing low amplitude and usually no diastolic flow (Fig. 4 B). Placing the sample on the medial anterior ovarian parts, signals were recorded in 67% (39/58) of cases.

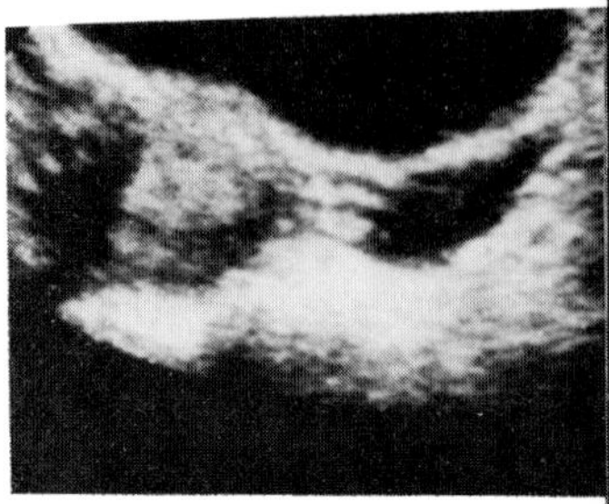

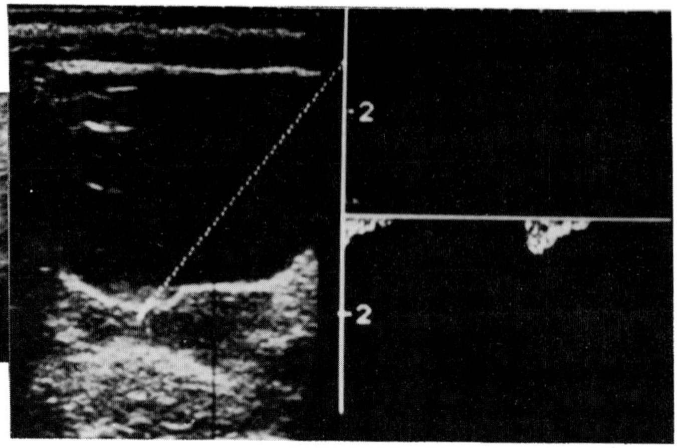

Fig. 4 A   Fig. 4 B

Fig. 4 A - Thin vessels originating at the upper part of the uterus and reaching left ovary believed to be terminal branches of the uterine artery.

Fig. 4 B - Waveforms obtained from ovarian ramus of the uterine artery (right) and sample position (left).

Scanning the lateral uterine wall at the level of uterine isthmus, a different type of waveform was recognized in 81% (47/58) of cases (Fig. 5). Regarding its anatomical position these vessels were supposed to be uterine arteries.

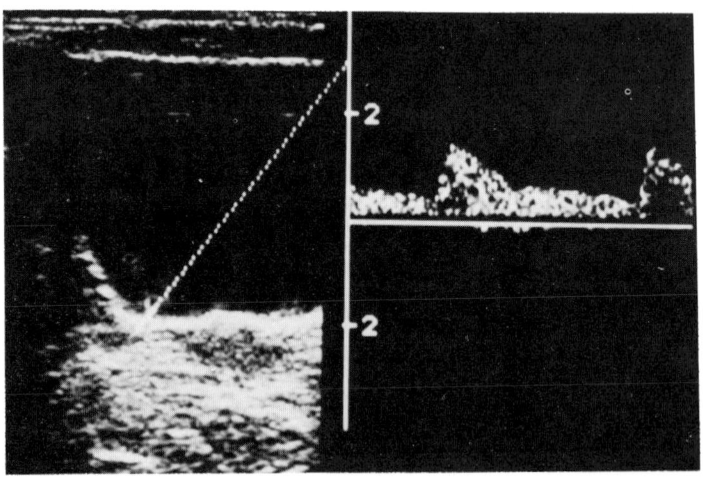

Fig. 5 - Low pulsatility waveform with marked diastolic flow (right) is characteristic for uterine artery.

DISCUSSION

Using our new method it was possible to visualize ovarian as well as the iliac vessels and to obtain a clear Doppler signal. This enables both qualitative and quantitative assessments of the blood flow in large vessels as the iliac arteries, where the errors in estimation of vessel diameter remain in acceptable range. According to Clark (12), turbulent flow effects which characterise small arterial plaque die out about 9 vessel diameters downstream from a stenosis. Employing our technique it is possible to improve diagnostic accuracy of ultrasound, recognizing the disease of aorto-iliac segment in female and most probably in male patients (13). The signals obtained from ovarian arteries and terminal branches of uterine arteries are in agreement with animal and hystological studies which suggested different organization of ovarian circulation during life (14). In the group of young healthy volunteers below the age of 20 it was not possible to obtain a signal from the ovarian ramus, but only a signal from the ovarian arteries was recognized almost regularly. At this age the ovarian blood supply depends mostly on the ovarian arteries. We found waveforms from both vessels showing characteristics of turbulent flow with small or no diastolic flow. Nimura et al. have reported that the flow patterns of the hepatic, splenic and both renal arteries exhibited a pattern of sustained flow throught one pulse period. These characteristics may be specific features of the arteries which perfuse parenchymatosus organs (15). We have recognized the same waveform of the ovarian arteries in approximately 50% of the cases. When using standard methods of analysis, the main problem was to interprete the second type of the signal we obtained. Failure in recognizing diastolic flow can occure due to increased vessel resistance or insuffitient technique of examination.

In vitro studies should be performed in an attempt to define the influence of changes in blood flow in the small vessels to waveforms characteristics (16).

It is our belief that this technique has a great potential and could provide additional data for better evaluation of normal and disturbed ovarian function.

REFERENCES

1. Johnston KW, Taraschuk I (1976) Validation of the role of pulsatility index in quantitation of the severity of peripheral arterial occlusive disease. Am J. Surg. 131:295-7
2. Fitzgerald DE, Drumm JE (1977) Non-invasive measurement of human fetal circulation using ultrasound: a new method. Br. Med. J. 2:1450-3
3. McCallum WD, Williams CS, Napel S, Daigle RE (1978) Fetal blood velocity waveforms. Am J Obstet Gynaecol, 132:425-9
4. Gill RW (1979) Pulsed Doppler with B-mode imaging for quantitative blood flow measurement. Ultrasound Med Biol, 5:223-9
5. Eik-Nes SH, Brubakk AO, Ulstein M (1980) Measurement of human fetal blood flow. Br Med J, 280:283-5
6. Griffin D, Bilardo K, Diaz-Recasens J, Teague MJ, Campbell S (1983) The measurement of human fetal blood flow with linear array pulsed Doppler duplex. Eur J Obstet Gynecol Reprod Biol 26:426-30
7. Campbell S, Diaz-Recasens J, Griffin DR, et al. (1983)New Doppler technique for assessing uteroplacental blood flow. Lancet, I:675-7
8. Kratochwil A, Urban G, Friedrich F (1972) Ultrasonic tomography of the ovaries. Ann Chirur Gynaec Fenniae, 6:211-4
9. Hackelöer BJ, Nitschke-Dabelstein S (1980) Ovarian imaging by ultrasound: An attempt to define a reference plane. J Clin Ultrasound 9:275-80
10. Hackelöer BJ (1984) The role of ultrasound in female infertility management. Ultrasound Med Biol 10:35-50
11. Funduk-Kurjak B, Kurjak A (1982) Ultrasound monitoring of follicular maturation and ovulation in normal menstrual cycle and in ovulation induction. Acta Obstet Gynecol Scand 61:329-31
12. Clark C (1980) The propagation of turbulence produced by a stenosis. J Biomechanics 13:591-604
13. Walton L, Martin TRP, Collins M (1984) Prospective assessment of the aorto-iliac segment by visual interpretation of frequency analysed Doppler waveforms: a comparison with arteriography. Ultrasound Med Biol 10:27-32
14. Watzka M. Harn und Geschlechtsapparat (1957) Berlin, Güttingen, Heilderberg: Springer Verlag 1957:123.
15. Nimura Y, Miyatake K, Kinoshita N, et al. (1983)In: Lerski RA, Morley P (eds) New approach to non-invasive assessment of blood flow in the major arteries in the abdomen by two-dimensional Doppler echography. Proceedings of the Third Meeting of the World Federation for Ultrasound in Medicine and Biology. Oxford:Pergamon Press, 447-51

Recent advances in ultrasound diagnosis 5. A. Kurjak, G. Kossoff, eds.

BLOOD FLOW IN FETAL AORTA, UMBILICAL ARTERY AND UTERINE ARTERY IN UTERO - PLACENTAL INSUFFICIENCY AND DURING LABOR

H. FENDEL

Department of Gynecology and Obstetrics of the RWTH Aachen
Director: Prof. Dr. med. H. Jung

INTRODUCTION

Our present knowledge about blood flow in the human fetus and the utero - placental unit has been gained by interpretation of the CTG or by animal studies using invasive methods. In the last decade the non invasive doppler technique has been developed to do blood flow measurements in fetal, in placental or in uterine vessels. GILL in Australia (1978) and EIK-NES with coworkers in Scandinavia (1981) have been one of the pioneers who did blood flow measurements with the pulsed doppler technique in pregnancy. In the last few years several authors described the changement of blood flow in vessels of small for date fetuses or in distressed fetuses and in uterine vessels in cases of an uteroplacental insufficiency (CAMPBELL,GRIFFIN 1983; JOUPILLA, KIRKINEN 1984; MARSAL et al. 1985).

The blood flow measurement by the pulsed doppler method in the fetal aorta and umbilical vessels is more or less accepted; but the blood flow measurement in uterine arteries, described by CAMPBELL, is still discussed.

To answer the question if the fetal distress or the uteroplacental insufficiency has to bee seen in a changement of a blood flow in uterine vessels,the dopplershift waveforms of the fetal aorta and the umbilical artery are compared with the dopplershift waveforms of uterine arteries.

METHOD

Pelvic vessels can be found on the lateral uterine wall. The bifurcation of the common iliac artery in external and internal iliac artery has to be identified (Fig. 1). The doppler profil which is found in the external iliac artery shows a high pulsatility with a reverse flow. The doppler profil in the internal iliac artery hasn't any reverse flow and the pulsatility is lower. If the doppler probe is directed from cranial to these vessels the flow goes away from the doppler probe in caudal direction. Cranial and more ventral to the external iliac artery there are very thin vessels (2-3 mm) nearly horizontal to the skin surface. Directing the doppler probe on these vessels there are very high shifted doppler waveform with a low pulsatility and the blood flow is going forwards (cranial) the doppler probe. The high dopplershift waveforms with the low pulsatility proves that the blood is pressed in these vessels with a high speed and that these vessels supply a vascular system with a low resistance. CAMPBELL believes that these vessels are the arcuate arteries.

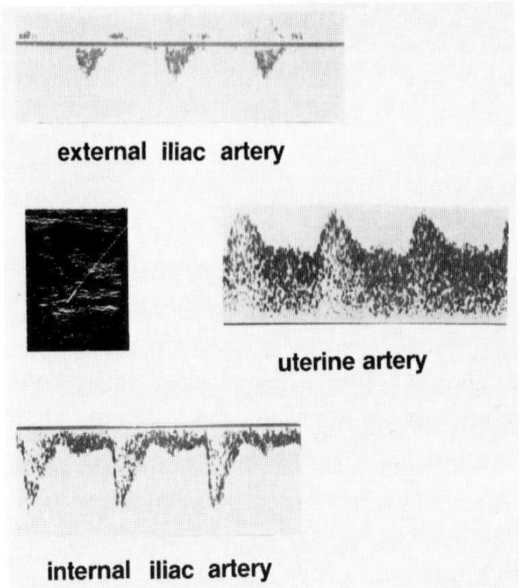

Fig. 1: Sonogram of the lateral pelvic wall with the large pelvic vessels and doppler-sonograms of the external iliac artery, the internal iliac artery and an uterine artery.

The typical dopplershift of the fetal aorta in a normal pregnancy shows a high pulsatility with a high systolic puls and a positive diastolic shift (Fig.2). In the umbilical artery a lower systolic puls changes to diastolic shift without visible incision between systole and diastole. The dopplershift of the uterine arteries with a low pulsatility indicates nearly a constant blood flow during the cardiac cycle. In placental insufficiency mainly the diastolic flow is changed. In a mild form of placental insufficiency the diastolic flow in the fetal aorta is decreased. In a severe form of placental insufficiency there isn't any diastolic flow visible at the end of the diastole. The similar changement can be found in the umbilical artery if there isn't any enddiastolic shift detectable there must be an increased resistance in the placental vascular bed. The reduction of the diastolic shifts in the doppler profile of uterine arteries can also be observed in uteroplacental insufficiency or in an increasment of uterine muscle activity for example during labor. In severe EPH-Gestosis the diastolic shift becomes very low, there is always a decreasement in the early diastole.

RESULTS AND DISCUSSION

The combination of all described doppler profils in the different vessels are possible. The normal dopplershift in the fetal aorta, umbilical artery and uterine artery indicates a well healthy fetus (Fig.3). The doppler measurement was done 1 week before delivery. The fetus was delivered spontaneously with a normal birth weight. The CTG is normal with a broad oscillation and accelerations.

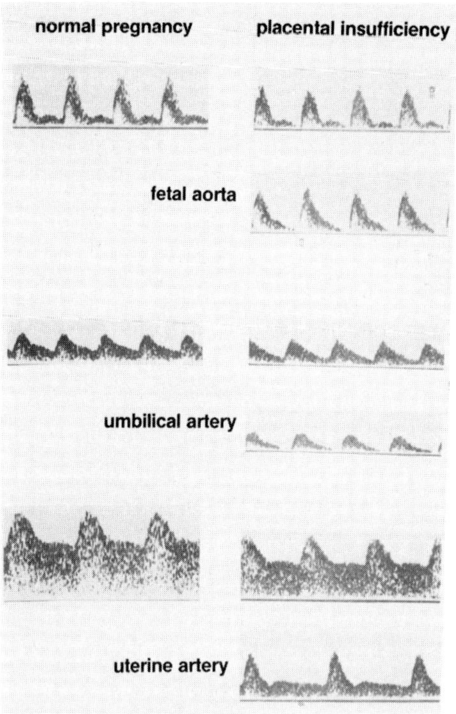

Fig.2: Dopplershift waveforms of fetal aorta, umbilical artery and uterine artery in normal pregnancy and in placental insufficiency.

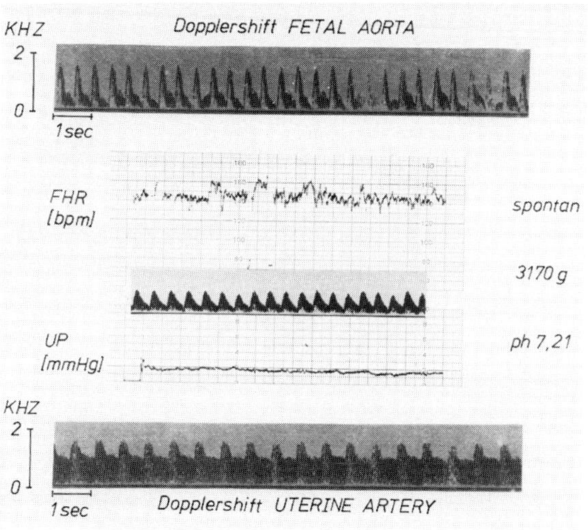

Fig.3: Normal dopplershift waveforms of fetal aorta, umbilical artery and uterine artery with normal CTG.

The decreasement of the diastolic shift in the fetal aorta,in the umbilical artery and in the uterine artery indicates an increased resistance in the fetus and in the uteroplacental unit (Fig.4). The fetal heart-rate is silent with a mild tachycardia. This fetus had to be delivered by cesarean section in the 36 week, because of an imminent asphyxia. The mother suffered from a severe EPH-Gestosis.

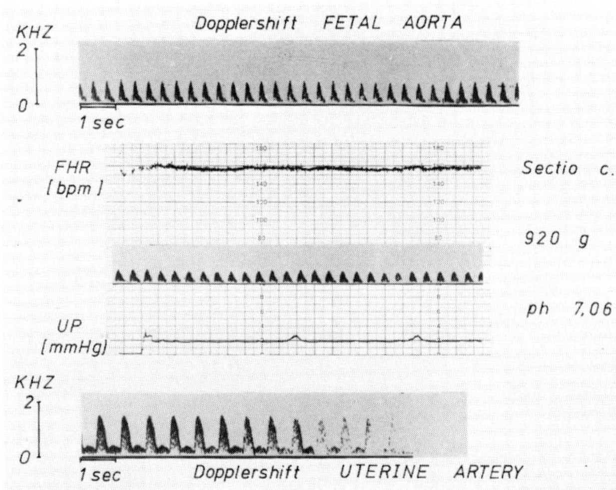

Fig.4: Decreased diastolic dopplershift in fetal aorta,umbilical artery and uterine artery because of severe placental insufficiency with silent fetal heart-rate.

The next case shows a reduction of the diastolic shift in the uterine artery with the typical dicrotic knodge in the early diastole in severe EPH-Gestosis (Fig.5). The mother suffered from a severe EPH-Gestosis. The dopplershift of the umbilical artery looks normally. The dopplershift of the fetal aorta shows an increased systolic shift, because of betamimetic therapy in preterm labor. The diastolic shift is normal in relation to the breathing movement of the fetus.The fetal heart-rate has a normal oscillation with a mild tachycardia because of betamimetic therapy. This fetus was born in the 35 week with 1.500 g spontaneously suffering from a compensated placental insufficiency.

A normal dopplershift of uterine artery with a reduced diastolic dopplershift in fetal aorta and umbilical artery is demonstrated in Fig.6. Blood flow measurements were done 5 hours before cesarean section because of an imminent asphyxia An increased resistance in fetal aorta and umbilical artery indicated a placental insufficiency of this small for date fetus.

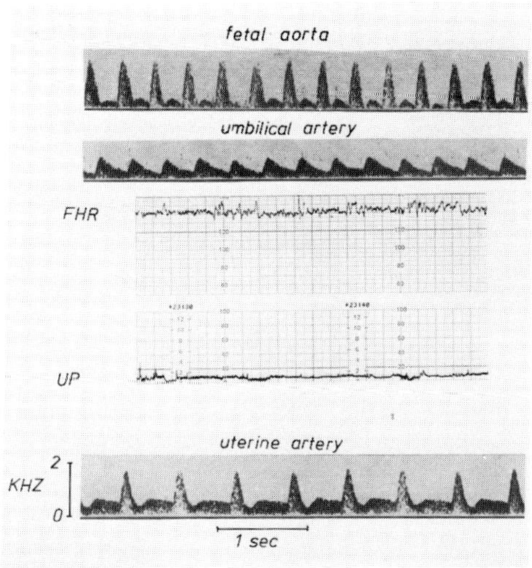

Fig.5: Normal dopplershift waveform in fetal aorta and umbilical artery and pathological dopplershift waveform in uterine artery because of EPH-Gestosis.

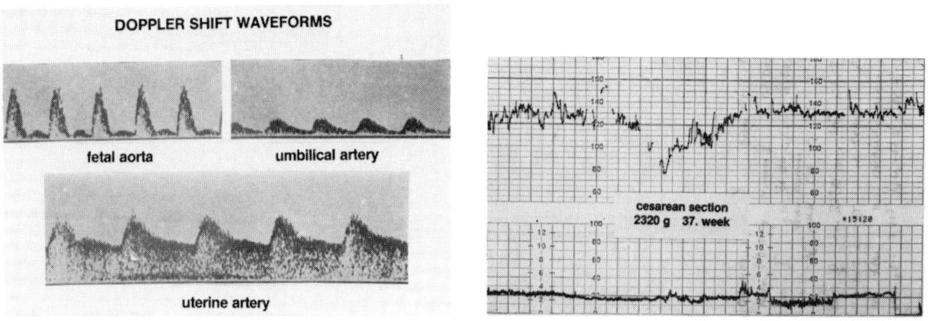

Fig.6: Decreased diastolic shift in fetal aorta and umbilical artery and a normal uterine artery dopplershift indicating an increased resistance in fetal aorta and umbilical artery because of placental insufficiency.

An abnormal dopplershift in the fetal aorta with a normal dopplershift in the uterine and umbilical artery is demonstrated in Fig.7. This case was recorded in the begining labor. The CTG shows variable decelerations. Nearly no diastolic shift is seen in the dopplershift waveform of the fetal aorta. This indicates an increased resistance in this vessel. Because of the normal diastolic shift in the umbilical artery the increasement of the resistance in the fetal aorta derives from the fetus itself.About 50 percent of the aortic flow volume goes back to the placental vascular bed and the remaining 50 percent of aortic blood flow volume is going to the peripheral vascular bed of the fetus. This small for date fetus had an increased resistance in his peripheral vascular system. The blood flow to the placenta in an umbilical artery was normal without an increased resistance So this small for date fetus was born spontaneously after 9 hours labor with a normal pH of the umbilical artery and a good apgar-score.

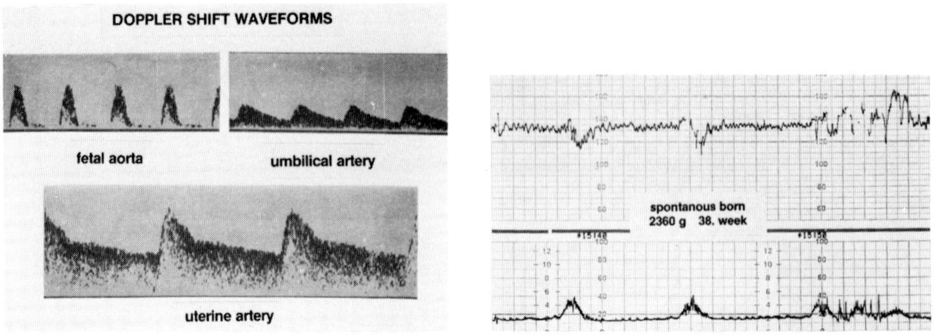

Fig.7: An abnormal dopplershift waveform of fetal aorta with a normal waveform of umbilical artery and uterine artery indicating a compensated placental insufficiency.

An example of a severe EPH-Gestosis with placental insufficiency is demonstrated in Fig.8. The enddiastolic shift in the waveform of the fetal aorta and umbilical artery is not visible and the pulsatility of the dopplershift waveform of uterine artery is increased. The diastolic dopplershift shows the typical dicrotic knodge in the beginning. Because of late decelerations this fetus had to be delivered by cesarean section.

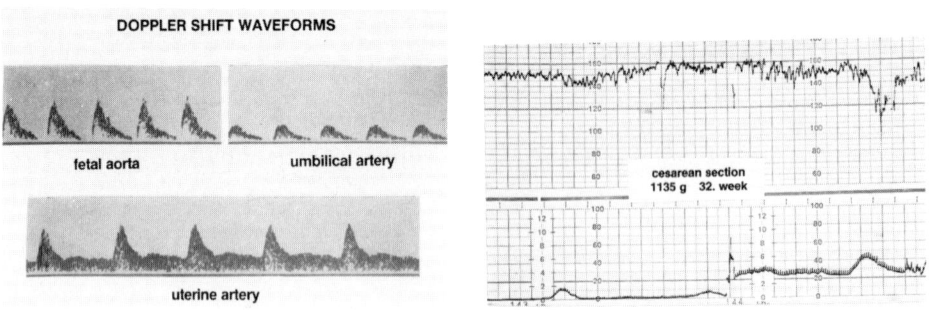

Fig.8: Pathological dopplershift waveforms of fetal aorta umbilical artery and uterine artery indicating an imminent asphyxia.

Comparing the values of the mean blood velocity in the fetal aorta of small for date fetuses in placental insufficiency with a value of normal weighted fetuses showed a significant difference (Tab.1). The difference of the mean blood velocity in the umbilical artery was not significant. In normal developed pregnancies we calculated a mean blood velocity of 58 cm/sec in uterine arteries. The mean blood velocity of 42 cm/sec in placental insufficiencies was significantly lower.

Mean blood velocity in fetal aorta,umbilical artery and uterine artery

Tab. 1

	V mean [cm/sec]		
	fetal aorta	umbilical artery	uterine artery
Placental insufficiency	28 ± 5 n 18	29 ± 5 n 7	42 ± 18 n 15
Normal pregnancy	33 ± 5 n 202	32 ± 7 n 66	58 ± 14 n 148
	$p < 0,001$	$p < 0,247$	$p < 0,000$

BLOOD FLOW DURING LABOR.

During labor blood flow is changed in the uterine arteries which can be seen by doppler measurement easyly. A Contraction reduces the diastolic and less the systolic dopplershift in uterine arteries (Fig.9). The fetus answers the decrease of the blood supply with an acceleration.

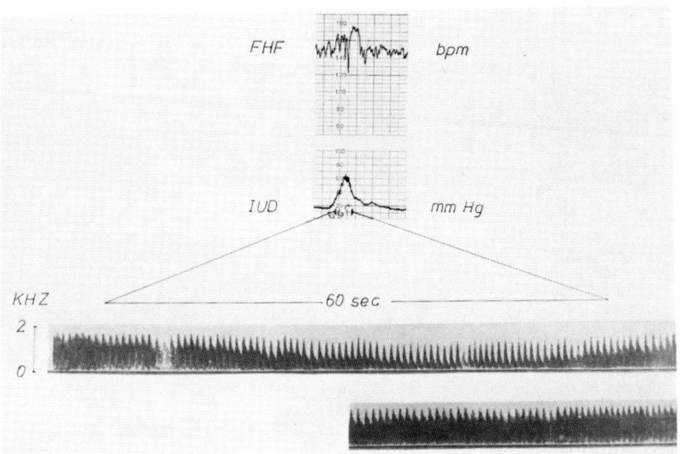

Fig.9: Dopplershift waveform of uterine artery during a mild contraction with the corresponding CTG.

A stronger contraction takes off completly the diastolic shift and the systolic shift is reduced to about 60 % of its value before the contraction (Fig.10). The fetus answers this strong contraction with an early deceleration. The short reduction of blood flow in the placenta leads to a reduction of oxygen which is seen in a decrease of the fetal heart-rate.

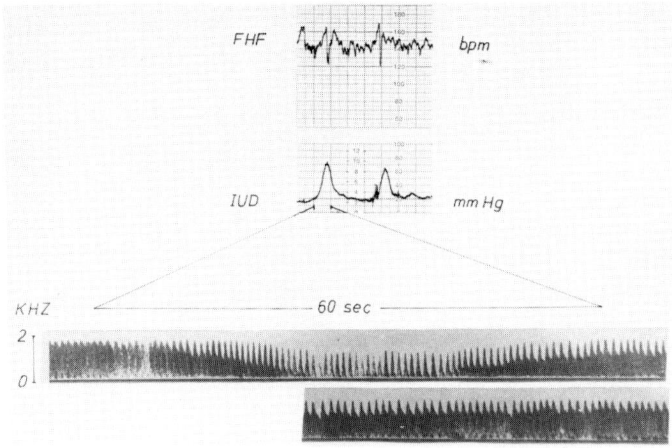

Fig.10: Dopplershift waveform of a uterine artery during a stronger contraction with the corresponding CTG.

During a double contraction (Fig.11) there isn't any diastolic dopplershift detectable in the uterine artery. This long lasting reduction of oxygen supply to the placental vascular bed is answered by the fetus with a broad late deceleration.

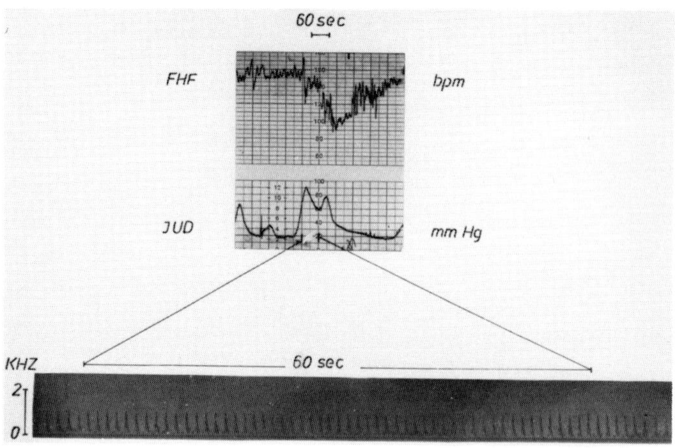

Fig.11: Dopplershift waveform of the uterine artery during a double contraction with late deceleration.

In 30 cases the blood velocity in uterine arteries was compared before and during contraction (Tab.2). The peak systolic velocity changed from 117 cm/sec to 99 cm/sec during contraction. This difference was not significant. But comparing the mean velocity there was a significant reduction from 55 cm/sec before contraction to 30 cm/sec during contraction. This prooves that the blood flow is reduced in uterine arteries during labor periodically and partly. But there isn't a complete interruption of blood flow in uterine arteries during contraction.

Blood velocity in uterine arteries during labor

n 30	V max cm /sec	V mean cm /sec
Before Contraction	**117** ± 22	**55** ± 18
During Contraction	**99** ± 23	**30** ± 14

Tab. 2

The blood flow in fetal decending aorta is not influenced in normal labor (Fig.12). Comparing the dopplershifts of the decending aorta before contraction and during contraction the waveform are similar, especially the diastolic shift is not altered because of the contraction. This was shown also by other authors like STEWART (1978) and MARSAL (1984).

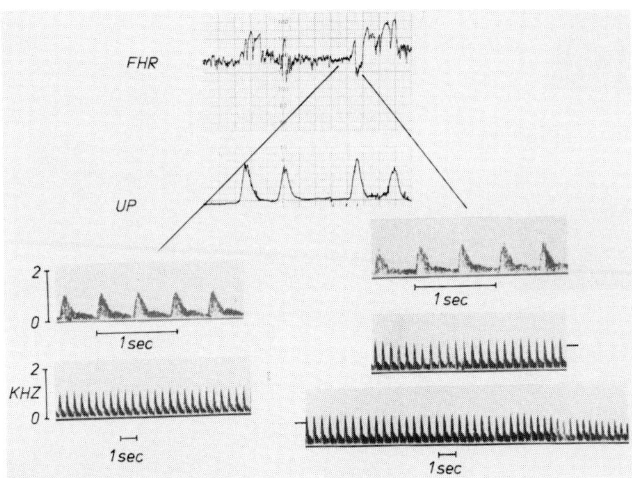

Fig.12: Dopplershift waveform of fetal aorta before and during contraction in normal labor.

When the CTG becomes pathologically with a silent heart-rate and with decelerations the doppler waveform of the fetal decending aorta is changed during contraction (Fig.13). Before the contraction the doppler waveform has it's normal pattern. During the contraction in the deceleration phase it is reduced in the diastolic period. In the acceleration phase the dopplershift increases again with a positive diastolic shift.

If the diastolic shift is heardly visible or completly undectable an increased resistance in the fetal aorta is indicated. It can be observed in an imminent asphyxia (Fig.14). This case was studied just before delivery by cesarean section because of a placental bleeding.

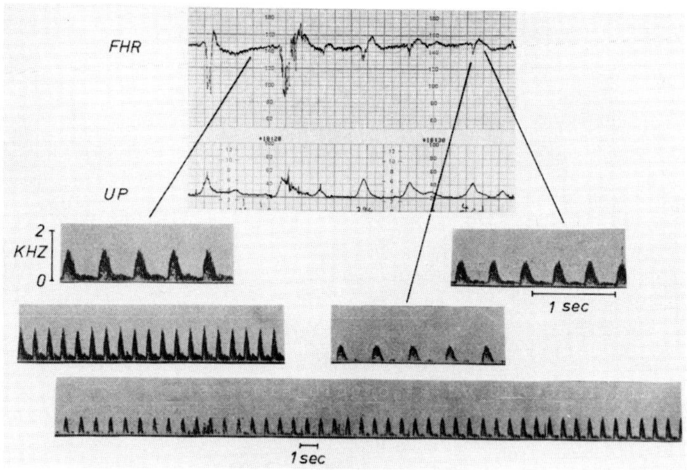

Fig.13: Dopplershift waveform of fetal aorta before and during contraction in pathological labor with silent fetal heart-rate and decelerations.

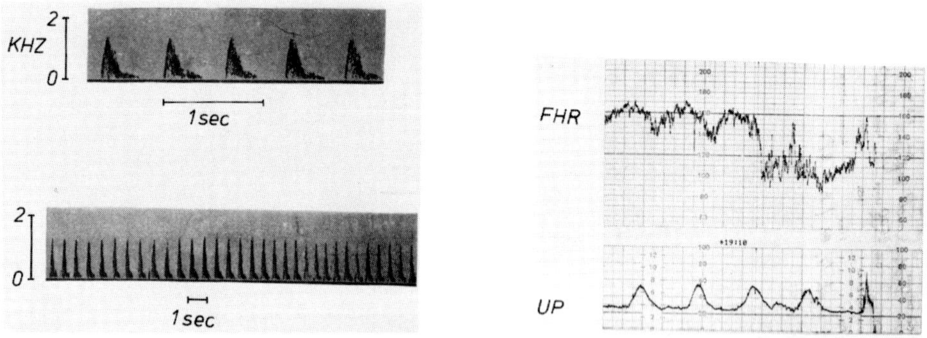

Fig.14: Dopplershift waveform of fetal aorta in pathological labor during bradycardia.

CONCLUSION

The dopplershift waveforms of fetal aorta,umbilical artery and uterine artery give a clear view regarding the fetal situation in the last trimester of pregnancy. In uteroplacental insufficiency with small for date fetuses the blood flow velocity is reduced in the fetal decending aorta and in the uterine artery. An increase of the vessel resistance is seen in the diastolic shift. The reduction of diastolic shift in the fetal aorta,the umbilical artery and the uterine artery is found in severe placental insufficiency mainly in EPH-Gestosis. Reduction of diastolic shift in fetal aorta but a normal dopplershift in umbilical and uterine artery indicates a compensated placental insufficiency with a small for date fetus. Normal blood flow in the fetal aorta and umbilical artery and reduced blood flow in the uterine arteries is found in EPH-Gestosis with a compensated placental insufficiency.

Blood flow in uterine arteries changes during contractions. The mean blood velocity is reduced significantly. In normal labor there isn't seen any change in fetal aortic dopplershifts,but in fetal imminent asphyxia the diastolic shift in the decending aorta is reduced or interrupted completely.

REFERENCES

1. CAMPBELL,S., D.R.GRIFFIN, J.M.J. DIAZ-RECASENS, T.E. COHEN -OVERBEEK, K. WILSON, M.J. TEAK: New doppler technique for assessing uteroplacental blood flow. The Lancet (1983) 675-677
2. EIK-NES, St.H., K. MARSAL, K. KRISTOFFERSEN, E. VERNERSSON: Non-invasive Messung des fetalen Blutstromes mittels Ultraschall. Ultraschall 2 (1981) 226-231
3. GILL, R.W.: Quantitative blood flow measurement in deeplying vessels using pulsed doppler with the octoson. In: Ultrasound in Medicine, Vol. 4, (1978) 341-348.
4. JOUPPILA, P.and KIRKINEN, P.: Increased vasculare resistance in the decending aorta of the human fetus in hypoxia. British Journal of Obstetrics and Gynecology (1984) 91, 853-856
5. MARSAL,K., A. LINDBLAD, G. LINGMAN and Sh. EIK-NES: Blood flow in the fetal decending aorta; intrinsic factors affecting fetal blood flow, i.e. fetal breathing movements and cardiac arrhythmia. Ultrasound in Medicine & Biol (1984)
6. STEWART, B., J. DRUMM, D.E. FITZGERALD and N.M. DUIGNON: Fetal blood velocity waveforms in uncomplicated labor. British Journal of Obstetrics and Gynecology (1978) 88, 865-869

Dr. med. H. Fendel, Abteilung Gynäkologie und Geburtshilfe der Medizin. Einrichtungen der RWTH Aachen, Pauwelsstr. o.Nr., D - 5100 Aachen

Recent advances in ultrasound diagnosis 5. A. Kurjak, G. Kossoff, eds.

PRENATAL TREATMENT OF FETAL CARDIAC ARRHYTHMIAS

J.W. WLADIMIROFF AND P.A. STEWART
Department of Obstetrics and Gynaecology, Academic Hospital Rotterdam-Dijkzigt, Erasmus University Rotterdam, Dr. Molewaterplein 40, 3015 GD Rotterdam (The Netherlands)

INTRODUCTION

Fetal cardiac arrhythmias are usually first suspected on the basis of auscultatory findings during routine pregnancy examination. Due to improved ultrasonic equipment, a more accurate diagnosis of the type of arrhythmia can be made, associated problems e.g. structural cardiac defects and cardiac compromise can be recognized and the effect of intrauterine treatment schedules closely monitored. The success of intrauterine therapy depends first and foremost on accurate intrauterine diagnosis. Until now intrauterine therapy for fetal cardiac arrhythmias has remained almost entirely restricted to pharmacologic interventions.

A basic issue in any intrauterine intervention is the question as to whether the recognized abnormality represents the only problem. Frequently, other organ systems are affected or an abnormal karyotype may be present. This may result in intrauterine intervention in an infant with unrecognized multiple congenital abnormalities. In general the decision to embark on intrauterine treatment of fetal arrhythmia depends on:
a. the type of arrhythmia present; b. the nature and seriousness of associated cardiac defects (and abnormal karyotype); c. the gestational age; d. the presence or absence of congestive heart failure or fetal hydrops; e. the presence or absence of fetal distress and/or labour; f. the availability of appropriate neonatal pediatric cardiac facilities.

Most reported arrhythmias are disorders of rate and/or rhythm of atrial origin and, abnormalities of conduction. The most clinically significant fetal arrhythmias regarding incidence and prognosis are supraventricular tachyarrhythmias and complete atrioventricular block. These conditions represent the most frequent underlying cause for congestive heart failure in utero.

DATA FROM OUR OWN UNIT

Altogether 97 cardiac arrhythmias were referred, 14 of which demonstrated normal sinus rhythm at the time of ultrasound examination. Gestational age varied between 18 and 41 weeks (mean: 32 wks). Three types of arrhythmia were observed:
ectopic beats (n = 52), bradycardia (< 100 bpm, n = 13) and tachycardia

(> 180 bpm, n = 18). Table I represents 14 patients with cardiac arrhythmias associated with cardiac structural defects.

Table I. Reasons for referral, gestational age at the time of diagnosis, ultrasonic and postpartum findings, mode of delivery and fetal outcome in 14 patients with cardiac structural problems.

Case no; Type of arrhythmia	Ultrasonic findings	Postpartum findings	Mode of delivery; fetal outcome
1. 34 wk, SVE	Univentricular heart + coarctation; IUGR	Confirmed	vag; IUD
2. 36 wk, SVE	Obstructive f.o.; enlarged right heart size	Normal structure; enlarged right heart size	vag; good
3. 37 wk, SVE	Obstructive f.o.; enlarged right heart size	Normal structure; enlarged right heart size	vag; good
4. 30 wk, SVE	? thick IVS (incomplete exam)	PAVSD	vag; good
5. 31 wk, SVE	enlarged right heart size; ? coarct (abn tricuspid valve)	peripheral pulmonary stenosis	vag; good
6. 37 wk, 3^oA-V block	RA tumour	Confirmed	vag; good
7. 29 wk, 3^oA-V block	Complex CHD + ascites	Confirmed + asplenia	vag; IUD
8. 20 wk, 3^oA-V block	Complex CHD + ascites	Confirmed + asplenia	Terminated (22 wk)
9. 35 wk, 2^oA-V block	VSD (great vessels not seen)	TOF + trisomy 18	CS;† 48 hrs postpartum
10. 29 wk, 3^oA-V block	Complex CHD (47XYY)	Confirmed	vag; IUD

11. 27 wk, Wandering pacemaker	Complete AVSD	Confirmed	vag; good
12. 40 wk, Sinus bradycardia	Aortic stenosis (severe maternal obesity)	Pulmonary stenosis	vag; good awaiting surgery
13. 35 wk, PSVT	Obstructive f.o.; enlarged right heart size	Normal structure; enlarged right heart size	vag; good
14. 22 wk, PSVT	IUD	Hypoplastic LV + fibroelastosis	IUD

SVE = supraventricular stenosis
TOF = tetralogy of Fallot
IUGR = intrauterine growth retardation
f.o.= foramen ovale
IUD = intrauterine death
vag.= vaginal delivery
IVS = interventricular septum
RA = right atrium
PAVSD = partial atrioventricular septal defect.

Ectopic beats were nearly always supraventricular (SVE; n = 50) and frequently appeared to be blocked. Five patients (Table I) with SVE (9%) had associated CHD resulting in fetal death in one (no 1). In two cases a membranous structure at the level of the foramen ovale was established; in the remaining two pregnancies (nos 4 and 5), CHD was suspected but not precisely diagnosed. All these four pregnancies developed uneventfully and fetal outcome was good.

Bradyarrthythmia (Table I) was diagnosed as complete atrioventricular block in 7 cases, 2nd degree atrioventricular block in 2 cases, mild-sinus bradycardia in 2 cases and thought to represent a recurrence of the sick sinus syndrome in one fetus. In one patient with an irregular bradycardia and complete atrioventricular septal defect (no 11) a wandering pacemaker was diagnosed postnatally.

In 5 of our patients bradycardia was associated with maternal collagen disease, in one case maternal symptoms becoming apparent 3 months after the delivery. In 7 patients (54%) bradycardia was associated with CHD (Table I). Twice a CHD was suspected but not correctly defined (nos 9 and 12), in one case this was due to excessive maternal weight (104 kg), and advances gestation (40 wks). The perinatal mortality rate was 38%.
Tachycardia (Table I) was assessed as paroxysmal supraventricular tachycardia

(PSVT) with spontaneous resolution in the 32nd week op pregnancy in one case, PSVT with multiple supraventricular extrasystoles (SVE) in 1 case, paroxysmal atrial flutter with multiple SVE's in 3 cases, sinus tachycardia in 1 case and atrial flutter with variable atrioventricular conduction and paroxysms of normal sinus rhythm in one case. There were 5 cases of supraventricular tachycardia (SVT), one of which was found to be a Wolff-Parkinson-White syndrome (WPW) postnatally. Three cases had atrial flutter with variable atrioventricular conduction. One patient had a normal heart rate as demonstrated by cardiotocography, but M-mode echocardiography revealed atrial flutter with variable atrioventricular conduction. One patient had atrial flutter with 2:1 atrioventricular conduction. One patient had short bursts of atrial flutter, sustained periods of SVT and multiple SVE's. Associated CHD was only established in two cases (11%). The perinatal mortality rate in the tachyarrhythmia group was 22%.

TREATMENT OF FETAL ARRHYTHMIAS

Attention will be focused on supraventricular tachyarrthythmias, since it is only this group of cardiac arrhythmias which is subject to prenatal treatment.

Tachyarrhythmias are almost exclusively of supraventricular origin. The most frequent observed tachyarrhythmia is paroxysmal supraventricular tachycardia (SVT) with heart rates above 180 bpm, often above 200-220 bpm and usually abrupt onset and termination. Atrial flutter and atrial fibrilation (300-480 bpm) nearly always with varying degrees of A-V block, have been documented. Differentation of SVT from fetal sinus tachycardia may be aided by the sustained higher heart rate (generally greater than 200 bpm) and a lack of beat to beat variation of SVT.

The estimated incidence is from 1 in 10.000 to 1 in 25.000 but even these figures are probably an underestimate since many cases are asymptomatic and undiagnosed (1,2).

Supraventricular tachyarrhythmias may be associated with functional instability of the atrial muscle, congenital heart disease, cardiac tumour and cardiomyopathy (3,4). Lately increasing attention is being focused on possible intrauterine infections such as cytomegaly and Coxsackie B virus as a cause of supraventricular tachyarrhythmia. Amniocentesis for viral culturing is therefore indicated. A common association in the presence of atrial fibrillation is the Wolff-Parkinson-White syndrome (5). Conduction system defects have been established in a number of infants with intrauterine arrhythmias (6).

Intrauterine treatment of fetal tachyarrhythmias can be defined as transplacental (via the mother) administration of antiarrhythmic agents to the fetus with the object to normalize fetal heart rate and rhythm and to abolish associated cardiac compromise. The rationale of intrauterine therapy in fetal tachyarrhythmias is twofold:

a) Tachyarrhythmias are often not well tolerated by the fetus, resulting in cardiac compromise (2,7,8).

b) After birth, there is a threefold increase in output of each ventricle greatly increasing cardiac work in spite of the elimination of the placenta from the circulation.

Table II provides data on transplacental therapy in the management of supraventricular tachyarrhythmias from our own Unit.

We only observed normalization of heart rate, sometimes intermittently, in three patients (no 1, 4 and 6, Table II). The former may even have been coincidental since maternal serum level of digoxin was only 0.4 ng/ml (therapeutic range 0.5 to 1.5 ng/ml). The poor outcome in our material is probably determined by the advanced stage of fetal hydrops which existed at the time of intrauterine treatment, resulting in fetal or neonatal death in cases 4,5 and 6. Only in cases 2 and 3 successful neonatal conversion using digoxin was achieved. Finally, it is of interest that in the successful cases in Table II, there is no relationship between the dose of therapy and termination of tachyarrhythmia, which suggests that other factors are involved. We personally believe that in a number of tachyarrhythmias heart rate may have returned to normal independent of intrauterine treatment. Long term, i.e. 24 hour recordings of fetal tachyarrhythmias are needed to obtain a better insight into the paroxysms of these arrhythmias.

In case of failure of digoxin treatment, other antiarrhythmic drugs such as propranolol, procainamide, verapamil (isoptin) and even amiodarone have been used in an attempt to normalize fetal heart rate. In some instances combined treatment with digoxin and another drug was attempted (9-14) (Table II).

Verapamil was used by us in two patients with fetal atrial flutter and advanced fetal hydrops. In one case (no 4; Table II) cardioversion was achieved, but Doppler flow measurements in the fetal descending aorta revealed poor myocardial contraction force; a flat fetal CTG indicated fetal hypoxia. A Caesarian Section was performed at 29 weeks. Despite resuscitative measures, the infant died on day 2. In Case no 6. (Table II), a total of 5 antiarrhythmic drugs was subsequently given. Only following amiodarone treatment a normal heart rate was obtained. However, hydropic features became more prominent and Doppler flow measurement in the descending aorta clearly established poor myocardial contraction force. A Caesarian Section was performed at 31 weeks. Despite cardioversion, the infant died

Table II. Transplancental treatment of fetal tachyarrhythmias in our own Unit.

Pat. no; Age of detection of tachyarrhythmia	Dose and Mode of therapy; Termination of tachyarrhythmia	Mode of delivery and gestational age; Fetal outcome
1. 38 wk, atrial flutter + 2:1 A-V block	digoxin: IV 1.75 mg daily mat serum: 0.4 ng/ml Term: yes, < 48 hrs	38 wk, vag.; NSR
2. 31^{+} wk, SVT	digoxin: orally 0.5 mg daily mat serum: 1.0 - 1.6 ng/ml Term: no	38 wk, CS.; digoxin, NSR
3. 34 wk, atrial flutter + variable A-V block	digoxin: IV 1.25 mg daily, mat serum: 1.0 - 1.2 ng/ml Term: no (occasional NSR)	35^{+} wk, CS.; digoxin, NSR
4. 27^{+} wk, atrial flutter + 2:1 A-V block	a)digoxin: IV 1.25 mg daily, then 1.0 mg daily mat serum: 4.5 ng/ml Term: no	
	b)verapamil:IV 20mg over 20 min Term: yes, but cardiac com- promise, CTG: fetal hypoxia	29 wk, CS.; NSR, digoxin, † on day 2; microscopy: normal conduction system
5. 25 wk, atrial flutter + 2:1 A-V block	a)digoxin:IV 0.75 mg daily mat serum: 0.8 ng/ml Term: no b)procainamide: IV 1 gr, then 4 gr daily mat serum: 2.4 mg/L NAPA : 1.4 mg/L Term: no c)verapamil: IV 10 mg over 60 min Term: no, † 27 wk	27 wk, vag.; micro- scopy: normal con- duction system
6. 25^{+}wk, SVT	a)digoxin b)verapamil c)procainamide d)inderal Term: no e)amiodarone Term: yes, but worsening hydrops	31 wk, CS., NSR, digoxin,† on day 2 microscopy: normal conduction system

on day 2 due to extreme cardiac compromise. Amiodarone, a benzofuran derivative has shown to be an extremely effective treatment for infants and children with tachyarrhythmias resistant to conventional treatment. Its use during pregnancy has been limited by insufficient knowledge of maternal-fetal transfer and the documented adverse effects of excessive iodine (15). Amiodarone, 200 mg, contains approximately 75 mg of iodine within its structure. The precise fate of this large amount of iodine is uncertain (16). Iodine is known to be:

a) transferred rapidly across the placenta even against a concentration gradient,

b) concentrated in fetal thyroid from as early as 14 weeks and,

c) associated with neonatal goiter after as little as 12 mg of iodine is ingested (17).

The risk of such complications for the individual patient is unpredictable and a genetic predisposition has been suggested (Croors, 1975).

When a fetal tachyarrhythmia has been established obstetric management including intrauterine treatment will depend on fetal maturity (age), the presence or absence of associated fetal cardiac abnormalities and abnormal karyotype. Careful 2D real-time analysis of fetal cardiac anatomy should be carried out. In the presence of a structural defect amniocentesis for karyotyping should be performed, since in about 45% of structural cardiac defects an abnormal karyotype has been established (14). In case of an inoperable cardiac defect and/or abnormal karyotype surgical intervention should be avoided. Having ruled out a cardiac structural defect in the presence of fetal tachyarrhythmia the initiation of intrauterine treatment mainly depends on fetal lung maturity.

In case of adequate lung maturity intrauterine treatment is not indicated and the infant should be delivered. The mode of delivery depends on obstetric conditions such as cervical maturity, fetal lie etc. Monitoring of fetal heart rate and fetal acid-base status should be carried out.

In case of insufficient lung maturity, intrauterine treatment should be started. When intrauterine therapy is successful, obstetric management will not be different from that in uncomplicated pregnancies. Regular 2D real-time ultrasonic monitoring of the fetus for imminent signs of cardiac compromise should be carried out. Vaginal delivery at term should be aimed for, although monitoring of fetal heart rate and fetal acid-base status is advisable because of the stress of labour. When intrauterine treatment fails, one should differentiate between fetal tachyarrhythmia without and with cardiac compromise. In the absence of cardiac compromise, delivery should take place as soon as fetal lung maturity can be expected. The mode of delivery depends on obstetrical conditions such as cervical maturity, fetal lie etc. In case of vaginal delivery, monitoring of fetal heart rate and fetal acid-base status is mandatory. In the mean time regular 2D real-time ultrasonic monitoring of the fetus for imminent signs of cardiac compromise must be performed. In the presence of cardiac compromise, it may be prudent to deliver the patient by Caesarian Section as soon as fetal lung maturity has been established in order to avoid the superimposed stress of labour on an already compromised fetus. In some instances, despite intrauterine therapy, progression to congestive heart failure may be such that surgical intervention at an earlier stage is necessary.

Finally, all infants should be delivered in the vicinity of an Intensive Neonatal Care Unit under supervision of a Neonatologist together with a Pediatric Cardiologist, since even those infants who did well during labour may develop cardiac failure in the neonatal period.

CONCLUSIONS

Fetal tachyarrhythmia is often life-treatening. Aggressive treatment is necessary in the light of developing cardiac compromise and lung immaturity.

Transplacental therapy with digoxin is still considered a first-choice approach. In case of failure, a combination of digoxin and verapamil may be considered, digoxin combined with propranolol, procainamide or quinidine may attempted as a next step, whereas amiodarone should be a last resort until more information about its possible effects on the fetal thyroid has been obtained. A combination of verapamil and propranolol should be avoided because both are negative inotropic agents.

REFERENCES

1. Ramzin MS, Hammacher K, Hinselmann M (1974) In: Perinatal Medicine, 4th Europ Congr Prague. Thieme Publishers, Stuttgart
2. Schreiner RL, Hurwitz RA, Rosenfeld CR et al (1978) J Perinat Med 6:274
3. Wedemeyer AL, Breitveld V (1975) Am J Dis Childh 129:738
4. Pearl W (1977) Southern Med J 70:622
5. Belhassen B, Pauzner D, Blieden L (1982) Circulation 66:1124
6. Siew Yen Ho, Mortimer G, Anderson RH (1985) Br Heart J 53:158
7. Hedwall G (1973) Acta Pediatr Scand 62:550.
8. Valerius NH, Jacobson JR (1978) Acta Obstet Gynecol Scand 57:407
9. Wolff F, Breuker KH, Schlensker KM et al (1980) J Perinat Med 8:203
10. Dumesic DA, Silverman NH, Tobais S et al (1982) N Engl J Med 307:1128

11. Spinnato JA, Shaver DC, Flinn GS (1984) Obstet Gynecol 64:730

12. Allan ZD, Crawford DC, Anderson RH et al (1984) Clin Cardiol 7:467

13. Vintzileos NH, Jacobson JR (1978) Acta Obstet Gynecol Scand 57:407

14. Wladimiroff JW, Stewart PA, Sachs ES, Niermeijer MF (1985) Amer J Clin Genetics 21:285

15. Ginsburg J (1971) Annu Rev Pharmacol Toxical 11:387

16. Broekhuizen J, Laruel R, Sion R (1969) Arch Int Pharmacodyn Ther 177:340

17. Burrow GN (1975) In: Volpe R (ed) Clinics in Endocrinology and Metabolism. WB Saunders, London, pp 115

Recent advances in ultrasound diagnosis 5. A. Kurjak, G. Kossoff, eds.

BLOOD FLOW IN NORMAL AND HIGH RISK PREGNANCIES

VIŠNJA LATIN, ATTILA PÁL, ŽARKO ALFIREVIĆ, ASIM KURJAK
Ultrasonic Institute, University of Zagreb, Yugoslavia

INTRODUCTION

Any factor affecting uterine blood flow may adversely affect fetal condition. The regulatory mechanisms involved in uterine blood flow are still not understood, but it is known that high uterine blood flow is, at least, partly achieved by an increase in maternal cardiac output and a fall in uterine vascular resistance (1). It is believed that low uterine vascular resistance is the consequence of trophoblast invasion and hormonal influence (2,3).

Umbilical blood flow increases with gestational age and weight and is also dependent on the vascular resistance and pressure gradient driving blood from the descending aorta through the placenta and back to the inferior vena cava (1).

In normal pregnancy the uterine placental (4) and umbilical placental (5,6) circulations are high flow low resistance vascular beds in which the increasing volume flow has been attributed to a decrease in resistance and to pressure increase.

Changes in feto-placental perfusion caused by increased peripheral resistance are usually the consequence of impaired utero-placental perfusion, and therefore attention has been turned recently, to the study of uterine blood flow (7).

Doppler ultrasound provides unique, non-invasive and safe method of studying blood flow characteristics in both fetal placental circulations and the maternal arterial supply to the intervillous space (7).

An on-line spectrum analyser enables instantaneous presentation of Doppler signals in a visual display as the Doppler spectrum and analyses of flow velocity waveforms (FVW). The FVW is described by the change in maximum velocity with time, and the Doppler sonogram is a graphic represntation of the FVW.

The flow velocity is influenced by ejection systolic pulse, arterial wall compliance, blood stream inertia and downstream peripherial resistance (8,9). The main area of clinical interest in studies of FVW is the assessment of resistance to flow in the placental villous vascular bed, since in this bed resistance is the major determinant of flow (7,10).

The ratio of peak systole to end diastole (A/B ratio) (11), the ratio of the difference between peak systole and end diastole to peak systole (the resistance index) (12) and the ratio of the peak to trough (or reverse peak) to the mean deviation from baseline (the pulsatility index) (13) have been suggested as measures of the effect of resistance on the FVW. In this study the A/B ratio of fetal aorta, umbilical arteries and uterine arteries in normal and high risk pregnancies was studied.

MATERIAL AND METHODS

A Kranzbühler 8130 Duplex system Doppler machine was used for all blood flow mesurements. A 3.5 MHz linear array ultrasound imaging system was combined with a 2 MHz pulsed Doppler.

Flow velocity waveforms were studied in 63 normal and 34 complicated pregnancies from 30th week to term. The complications in high risk pregnancies are listed in Table 1. The majority of cases were pregnancies with mild gestosis (index 4-7) and only two were severe.

TABLE I

LIST OF COMPLICATED PREGNANCIES

Diagnosis	No. of patients
EPH gestosis	14
Suspected growth retardation	9
Diabetes mellitus	4
Rh iscimmunization	2
Cholostasis	2
Antepartum hemorrhage	2
Hyperthyreosis	1
Total	34

The women were examined in a semi-recumbent position and the uterus was scanned to identify fetal position and placental side. Fetal aorta, umbilical artery and arcuate artery on the placental and non-placental side were observed during the third trimester.

The A/B ratio in all of them was calculated.

The fetus was studied by orienting the transducer longitudinally to visualize the descendent part of the fetal aorta. The analyses were performed during the period of fetal apnea. Peak systole and end diastole were measured on the screen and A/B ratio was calculated according to the shown formula.

Recording of the umbilical artery is usually simple. The real time scanner was used to locate a loop of the umbilical cord, although the audible Doppler signal is readily heard and distinguished by ear from the fetal aorta and maternal vessels.

To find the arcuate artery the transducer was directed to the lateral pelvic side wall to identify the common iliac artery and its bifurcation, or directly onto the uterine wall to try to visualize the arcuate artery, or to find the typical audible sign. It is so specific that it cannot be confused with any other signal, because of its low pulsatility with high velocities in the diastole.

Gestational age was determined by a combination of clinical assessment and ultrasound examinations. Obtained values of A/B ratio in both groups of women were compared and studied.

RESULTS

TABLE II

OUTCOME OF PREGNANCY

	Apgar score $\geqslant 6$		Caesarian Section		Perinatal death	
	N	%	N	%	N	%
Normal pregnancy N=63	2	3.3	2	3.3	1	1.6
Complicated pregnancy N=34	4	11.8	6	17.6	0	-

In our group of normal pregnancies all babies were delivered after 38 weeks of gestation. Two of them (3.3%) had a low Apgar score and two were delivered by Caesarian section because of descendent umbilical cord and cephalopelvic disproportion. The baby born by vaginal breech delivery was severely hypoxic and died immediately after delivery.

In the high risk group pregnancies 11.8% of babies had a low Apgar score. In this group 6 CS were performed (17.6%) because of fetal condition (hypoxia), but no baby died.

Analysing FVW from the fetal aorta and umbilical artery no significant differencies in A/B ratio between normal and high risk pregnancies were obtained.

In normal pregnancies the A/B ratio values of the fetal aorta slightly decrease in the last trimester from 4.77 ± 1.08 at the begining of the third trimester to 4.16 ± 0.66 at the end of pregnancy. In complicated pregnancies the A/B ratio values in the same period were higher (5.00 ± 0.79 and 4.30 ± 1.36 respectively). There was no significant difference between A/B ratio values in normal and complicated pregnancies at 30-33, 34-37 and 38-41 weeks of gestation ($t=0.61$, $p > 0.1$ at 30-33 weeks; $t=0.61$, $p > 0.1$ at 34-37 weeks; $t=0.28$, $p > 0.1$ at 38-41 weeks) (Fig. 1).

FIGURE I
THE A/B RATIO (MV ± SD) IN FETAL AORTA
(NORMAL AND COMPLICATED PREGNANCIES)

	Weeks of gestation		
	30-33	34-37	38-41
A/B ratio in normal pregnancy N=63	4.77 ±1.08	4.35 ± 1.27	4.16 ± 0.66
A/B ratio in complicated pregnancy N=34	5.00 ± 0.79	4.63 ± 0.80	4.30 ± 1.36
t	0.61	0.61	0.28
p	> 0.1	>0.1	>0.1

Analysing data in umbilical artery FVW a decrease in A/B ratio in last trimester was obtained. In normal pregnancies at 30 weeks of gestation the A/B ratio was 2.45 ± 0.48 and at the end of pregnancy 2.01 ± 0.35. In high risk patients the obtained values were higher, but there was no significant difference between A/B ratio values in both investigated groups at 30-33, 34-37 and 38-41 weeks ($t= 1.61$, $p > 0.1$ at 30-33 weeks; $t= 0.08$, $p > 0.1$ at 34-37 weeks; $t= 0.36$, $p > 0.1$ at 38-41 weeks) (Fig. 2).

FIGURE
THE A/B RATIO (MV ± SD) IN UMBILICAL ARTERY
(NORMAL AND COMPLICATED PREGNANCIES)

	Weeks of gestation		
	30-33	34-37	38-41
A/B ratio in normal pregnancy N= 63	2.45 ± 0.48	2.18 ± 0.36	2.01 ± 0.35
A/B ratio in complicated pregnancy N= 34	2.83 ± 0.69	2.30 ± 0.52	2.06 ± 0.22
t	1.61	0.08	0.36
p	>0.1	>0.1	>0.1

In arcuate artery A/B ratio in normal pregnancy decreased from 30 to 40 weeks of gestation (1.52 ± 0.13 to 1.41 ± 0.09). In complicated pregnancies, however, an increase in A/B ratio values was found (1.55 ± 0.17 - 1.67 ± 0.23). There is a significant difference between A/B ratio values in normal and high risk pregnancies from 34 weeks onward ($t= 1.97$, $p>0.05$, $p<0.1$ at 34-37 weeks; $t= 4.59$, $p<0.01$ at 38-41 weeks) (Fig. 3).

FIGURE 3
THE A/B RATIO (MV ± SD) IN ARCUATE SRTERY
(NORMAL AND COMPLICATED PREGNANCIES)

	Weeks of gestation		
	30-33	34-37	38-41
A/B ratio in normal pregnancy N= 63	1.52 ± 0.13	1.43 ± 0.13	1.41 ± 0.09
A/B ratio in complicated pregnancy N= 34	1.55 ± 0.17	1.68 ± 0.20	1.67 ± 0.23
t	0.19	1.97	4.59
p	>0.1	>0.05 <0.1	<0.01

Both placental and nonplacental sides of the uterus were also investigated, and A/B ratio was calculated. It is interesting that in normal pregnancies there is a significant difference in A/B ratio between the two sides of the uterus from the 30th week of pregnancy to the end of pregnancy (t= 2.88, $p<0.01$ at 30-33 weeks; t= 3.07, $p<0.01$ at 34-37 weeks; t= 4.91, $p<0.01$ at 38-41 weeks (Fig. 4).

FIGURE 4
THE A/B RATIO (MV ± SD) IN ARCUATE ARTERIES ON PLACENTAL AND NONPLACENTAL SIDE IN NORMAL PREGNANCY

	Weeks of gestation		
	30-33	34-37	38-41
The A/B ratio on placental side N= 63	1.52 ± 0.13	1.43 ± 0.13	1.41 ± 0.09
The A/B ratio on nonplacental side N= 63	1.87 ± 0.32	1.61 ± 0.23	1.62 ± 0.15
t	2.88	3.07	4.91
p	< 0.01	<0.01	<0.01

In complicated pregnancies, however, no significant differences were found comparing A/B ratio values obtained on placental and nonplacental sides. (In all investigated periods $p>0.1$). (Fig. 5)

FIGURE 5
THE A/B RATIO IN ARCUATE ARTERIES ON PLACENTAL AND NONPLACENTAL SIDE IN COMPLICATED PREGNANCY

	Weeks of gestation		
	30-33	34-37	38-41
A/B ratio on placental side N= 34	1.55 ± 0.17	1.68 ± 0.20	1.67 ± 0.23
A/B ratio on nonplacental side N= 34	1.70 ± 0.22	1.83 ± 0.84	1.85 ± 0.36
t	1.21	0.39	1.30
p	>0.1	>0.1	>0.1

COMMENT

According to our results obtained from investigated vessels, the FVW in normal pregnancy showed high diastolic flow velocities. The A/B ratio decreased from 30 weeks to the end of pregnancy, slightly in the fetal aorta and umbilical artery and more pronounced in the arcuate artery. Low Apgar score in two cases and one neonatal death were not connected with complications of pregnancy which can affect fetal well-being. The complications occured in labour and were associated with management of labour.

In the high risk group, where a higher incidence of low Apgar score and Caesarian section were found, the complications were the direct consequence of pathology. In this group no significant differences in fetal circulation were found, comparing normal and high risk pregnancies. But in maternal circulation the A/B ratio was significantly higher in high risk pregnancies compared with normal pregnancies.

There is much speculation as to whether the fetus determines its placental and uteroplacental blood flow or the uteroplacental flow constrains the fetus (10). Also, it has not been clearly established in what part of fetal umbilical and maternal uterine circulations can the first disturbances be recognized, predicting fetal compromise.

According to our data the first sign of fetal compromise are disturbances in maternal circulation. Immediate influence on fetal blood flow was not observed, because these pathological changes obviously could not influence A/B ratio values. Using index profile after computer analyses will, perhaps, allow detection of abnormal changes in fetal circulation.

Analysing single cases we found a connection between high A/B ratio in the umbilical artery and fetal aorta and neonatal complications, but the number of these patients investigated at the time, was too small.

It is interesting that in normal pregnancies the significant differences in A/B ratio between the placental and nonplacental side were found. Similar differences were not observed in complicated pregnancies. This needs further investigation and comparison of these data with fetal outcome in a larger study group. We may be able to conclude that this parameter could be used as additional predictor of normal or complicated pregnancies during the first examination.

REFERENCES

1. Walsh SZ, Lind J (1978) In: Stave U (ed) The fetal circulation and its alteration and birth. Plenum Medical Book Co. New York, pp 129

2. Hamilton WJ, Boyd JD (1966) Trophoblast in human uteroplacental arteries. Nature 212: 906-908

3. Robertson WB, Brosens J, Dixen G (1975) Uteroplacental vascular pathology. European J. Obstet. Gynecol. and Reproductive Biology 5: 47-65

4. Eik-Nes SH, Brubakk HC, Ustein MK (1980) Measurement of human fetal blood flow. Br. Med. J. 280: 284

5. Rudolph AM, Heymann MA (1970) Circulation changes during growth in the fetal lamb. Circ. Res. 26: 289-99

6. Dawes GS (1968) Umbilical maternal placental and myometrial blood flow in fetal and neonatal physiology. Year Book Medical Publisher, Chicago 60-5

7. Griffin D, Cohen-Overbeek T, Campbell S (1983) Fetal and Uteroplacental Blood Flow. Clinics in Obstet. and Gynecol. 10: 565-602

8. MacDonald DA (1974) Blood flow in arteries. Edward Arnold Publishers Ltd. London 118-46

9. O'Rourke MF (1982) Vascular impedance in studies of arterial and cardiac function. Physiol. Rev. 62: 570-623

10. Trudinger BJ, Giles WB, Cook CM (1985) Flow velocity waveforms in the maternal uteroplacental and fetal umbilical placental circulations. Am. J. Obstet. Gynecol. 152: 155-160

11. Stuart B, Drumm J, Fitzgerald DE, Duigan NM (1980) Fetal blood flow velocity waveforms in normal pregnancy. Br. J. Obstet. Gynecol. 87: 780-785

12. Pourcelot L (1974) In: Perroneau (ed) Application cliniques de l'examen Doppler trannscutane, In Velocimetric ultrasonor Doppler P. Inserm 34: 213-240

Recent advances in ultrasound diagnosis 5. A. Kurjak, G. Kossoff, eds.

UTERINE ACTIVITY AND UMBILICAL BLOOD FLOW

ANTE KLOBUČAR, BRANKO RAJHVAJN and ASIM KURJAK

Ultrasonic Institute, "Dr Josip Kajfeš" Hospital
University of Zagreb, Yugoslavia

INTRODUCTION

Small-for-dates babies are still a problem for an obstetrician and pediatrician because these neonates have a fivefold increase in perinatal mortality in comparison with babies of normal weight (1). There are many factors which alone or combined may lead to the development of IUGR. The most important extrinisic factor affecting the placenta and leading to IUGR seems to be a decrease in uteroplacental blood flow. Recently, it was shown that there is strong correlation between decreased umbilical blood flow and IUGR (2,3,4). During intrauterine life the integrity of feto-placental circulatory system has the major responsibility of transporting the essential elements in their transfer from mother to the fetal tissues accross the placenta and bringing back to the placenta fetal catabolic products.

Uterine blood vessels carry arterial blood into placenta, and take venous blood out of it. As these vessels pass through myometrium, they are influenced by it. This myometrical muscle pressure especially influence the veins with thin muscle walls, and a low blood pressure. Therefore, this very influence is in the corelation with myometrical blood pressure.

It is supposed that myometrial activity in pregnancy may have a considerable influence on fetal blood flow through intervillous space, i.e. indirectly through umbilical vein. The correlation between uterine activity in pregnancy and fetal growth was examined.

MATERIAL AND METHODS

A group of 200 pregnant women from 32 to 40 weeks of gestation were examined. 100 of these pregnants had a completely normal uterine activity and normal pregnancy and they formed a control group. In the other group of 100 patients, a pathologic uterine activity was found. In all of them fetal blood flow in umbilical vein was measured according to the Eik-Nes method (4). The measurements of blood flow were performed on Toshiba-Sonolayer

SAL 50 A machines.

The activity of pregnant uterus was measured electromyographically on Medelec MS-6 machine, with filters adjusted for smooth muscles. That was recording and analysis of electronic activity of uterus. That activity was manifested by bursts of biopotentials of specific shape and duration. Using this technique six categories of recordings were defined. It should be emphasized, that there were no correlation between electric and mechanical activity of the whole uterus, up to a certain gestational age (7). Therefore, it was possible to follow and estimate these activities and record their premature occurance in a pathological pregnancy. The electromyographical examination was displayed in the Fig. 1.

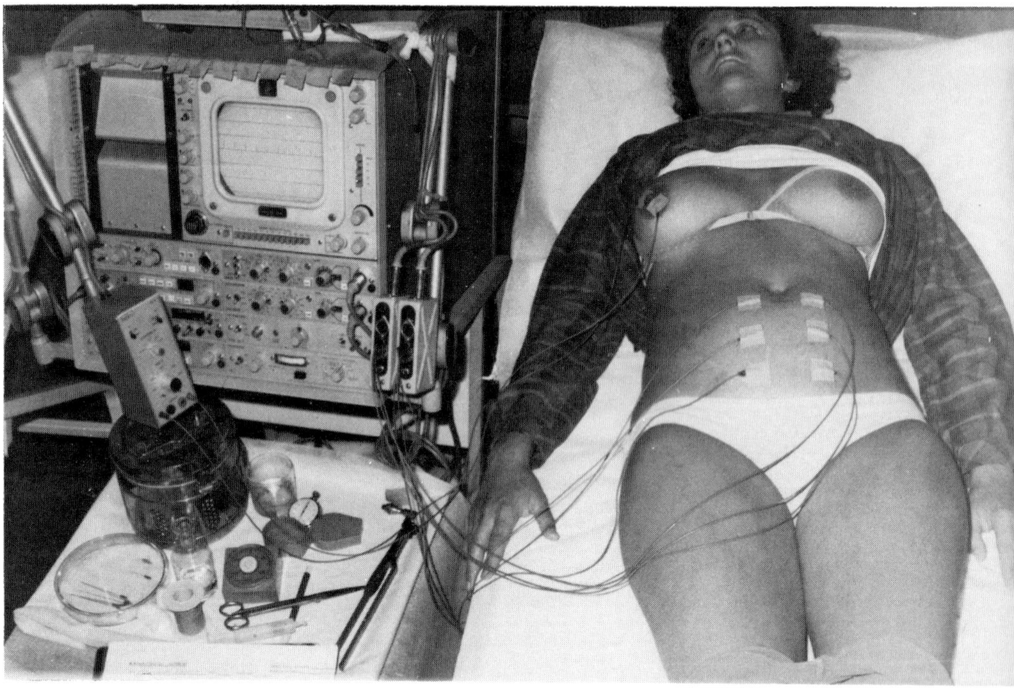

Fig. 1. Typical electromyographical examination in pregnancy combined with electrostimulation of mammilla

According to electromyographical finding uterine activity was devided in six groups. The features of each group are described in Table 1. During normal pregnancy, there is a characteristic asynchronization between electronic and mechanical activity of the uterus, while a synchronization takes place only immediately before the labor. In the first group we were not able to record any spontaneous or provoked uterine activity because it appears only in the normal pregnancy. Next four groups show slightly, medium, extremly, and potentially, sensibilized uterus and they are characteristic finding of premature pathological activity. This activity is recorded by train discharges of certain number of biopotentiales, with different duration and irregular occurance. Sometimes if there are fewer discharges, they are not correlated to the mechanical activity of the whole uterus. Extreme biopotentials with higher amplitudes in one discharge denote a transition phase towards synchronization and result in early labour. This group has phasic activity of the uterus because periods of electric activity are followed by periods of electric silence. This activity is called phasic or rhythmic activity of uterus. Clinically, it is sensibilized uterus, and in these women a treatened abortus or preterm labor can occur.

The uterine activity can be recorded as continuous discharges of biopotentials without pauses as well. Smooth muscles can keep the tense position without being rhythmically contracted. They can maintain the state of hypertonus without loosing much energy for that action (3). Electromyographicaly this uterine hypertonus is recorded by steady biopotential bursts of low amplitude. The duration of this tension can be long, and it can even be a characteristic of a particular pregnancy. The last group represents hypertonic status of the uterus in pregnancy. Classic tocolitics mainly have no influence upon such a condition, because it is mostly caused by activation of prostaglandin or histamine receptors.

Considering parity, patients were divided into primigravidas and multigravidas, and further to patients with male or female infants. Therefore, sex of fetuses was previously determined by ultrasound. The weight of fetus was estimated by ultrasound according to Kurjak-Breyer's method (8). The weight of the fetus of particular gestation age was compared with the standard one according to Thomson, and the blood flow findings were compared with the standard flow according to Rajhvajn (2), and with our own control group.

TABLE I

EMG: ASSESSMENT OF THE UTERINE ACTIVITY IN PREGNANCY

SPONTANEOUS ACTIVITY		PROVOKED ACTIVITY		ASSESSMENT
N° AP/10 min	AMPLITUDE	LATENT PHASE	TYPE OF REACTIVITY	
O	O	O	O	NORMAL PREGNANCY
$<$10 AP	500-1000 μV	$>$30 sec	I	SLIGHTLY SENSIBILIZED UTERUS
10 - 30 AP	500-2000 μV	$<$30 sec	II - III	MEDIUM SENSIBILIZED UTERUS
$>$30 AP	500-3500 μV	$<$15 sec	III - K	EXTREMELY SENSIBILIZED UTERUS
O	O	$<$15 sec	II - III	POTENTIALLY SENSIBILIZED UTERUS
CONTINUOUS MONOTONOUS DISCHARGES	to 1500 μV	O	O	HYPERTONUS

RESULTS

Altogether, 100 pregnant women with normal electromyographic finding of uterus, from 32 to 40 weeks of pregnancy, were investigated. These healthy women formed a control group. They gave birth to eutrophic newborns with normal growth development in pregnancy. There was none small-for-age newborn. Weight deviations in these fetuses from Thomson (9) and Rajhvajn's (2) standards, were minimal. 50 women with phasic activity of uterus from 32nd to 40th week of pregnancy, were investigated. Blood flow and electromyographic findings were afterwards examined once a week until the labor.

In primigravidas with male infants the average blood flow was 112 ± 11.1 ml/min/kg. In relation with the standard umbilical vein blood flow according to Rajhvajn (2) the deviation of the flow was minimal.Fetal weight minimally deviated from Thomson's weight standard. The average weight of this group was 3450 ± 291 g. All the newborns were eutrophic and healthy, except one small-for-age infant.

In primigravidas with female newborns, the average blood flow through umbilical fetal vein was 113,4 ± 11,2 ml/min/kg. Considering standard umbilical fetal flow according to Rajhvajn (2), there was a minimal deviation. Similarly the fetal weight, was slightly lower than that one according to Thomson. The average fetal weight was 3370 ± 104,5 g. There were no hypothrophic newborns in this group.

In multigravidas with male newborns, the average blood flow was 112,6 ± 13,1 ml/min/kg. Considering Rajhvajn's (2) and Thomson's (9) standards, the blood flow and fetal weight were slightly lower. The average weight was 3360 ± 138 g. There was one hypothrophic, smal--for-age infant, with a low umbilical vein blood flow.

In multigravidas with female newborns, the average umbilical vein blood flow was 111,6 ± 15,7 ml/min/kg. Fetal blood flow and weight did not significantly deviate from the standard one. The average weight of the newborns was 3270 ± 201,5 g. There were no hypothrophic cases at all.

50 pregnant women with hypertonic uterine activity from 32nd to 40th week of pregnancy were investigated. Umbilical vein blood flow and electromyographic finding of uterus were examined once a week during pregnancy until the labor.

In primigravidas with male newborns significant decrease of blood flow and the average fetal weight were observed. The average umbilical vein blood flow was 77,3 ± 26,3 ml/min/kg. According to Rajhvajn's standard (2), it was significantly lower (Fig. 2).

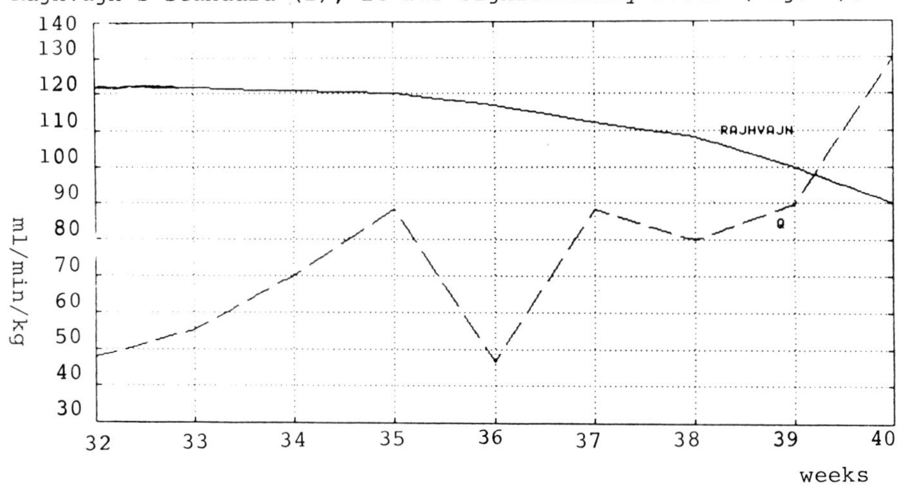

Fig. 2. Fetal umbilical blood flow and hypertonic uterine activity in primigravidas with male newborn infants

Average weight of these children was 2710 $\pm$ 368 g. There were 37,5 % of hypothrophic children with the weight below the 5th percentile for gestational age.

In primigravidas with female infants, the blood flow was low i.e. 76,8 $\pm$ 23,8 ml/min/kg (Fig. 3). The average weight of fetuses of this group was significantly lower than the standard one according to Thomson (9). The average birth weight was 3000$\pm$342 g. There were 20% hypothrophic children with weight below the 5th percentile for gestational age.

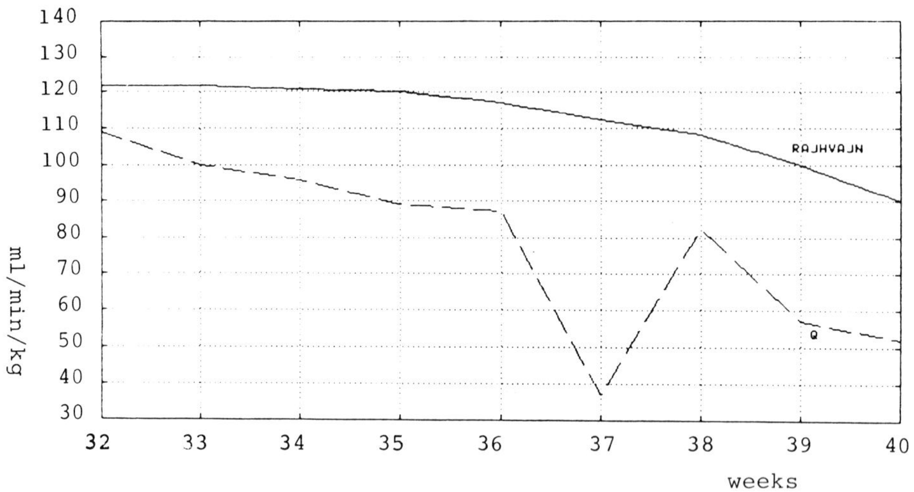

Fig. 3. Fetal umbilical blood flow and hypertonic uterine activity in primigravidas with female infants

In multigravidas with male newborns the average blood flow in fetal umbilical vein was 72,53 $\pm$ 20,1 ml/min/kg. Umbilical vein blood flow was permanently significantly lower than the standard one according to Rajhvajn (2) (Fig. 4). The average fetal weight, considering Thomson's (9) standard, was significantly lower, too. The average birth weight was 3050 $\pm$ 129,8 g. There were 25 % of hypothrophic children with weight below the 5th percentile for gestational age.

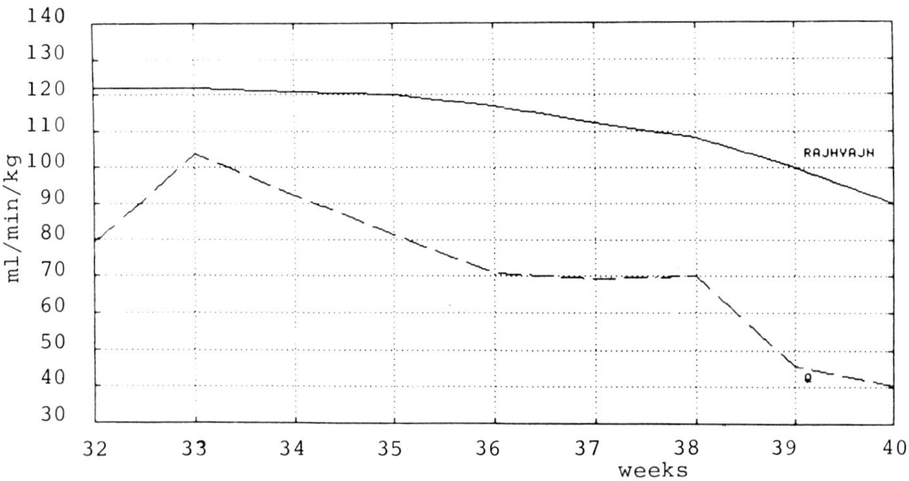

Fig. 4. Fetal umbilical blood flow and hypertonic uterine activity in multigravidas with male infants

In multigravidas with female infants the average blood flow in umbilical vein of fetus was 72,9 ± 24 ml/min/kg. The flow and weight were significantly lower than Rajhvajn's (2) standard (Fig. 5). The average birth weight was 2900 ± 176 g. Those were low-birth-rate newborns, without hypothrophic ones, below the 5th percentile in weight for gestational age (0%).

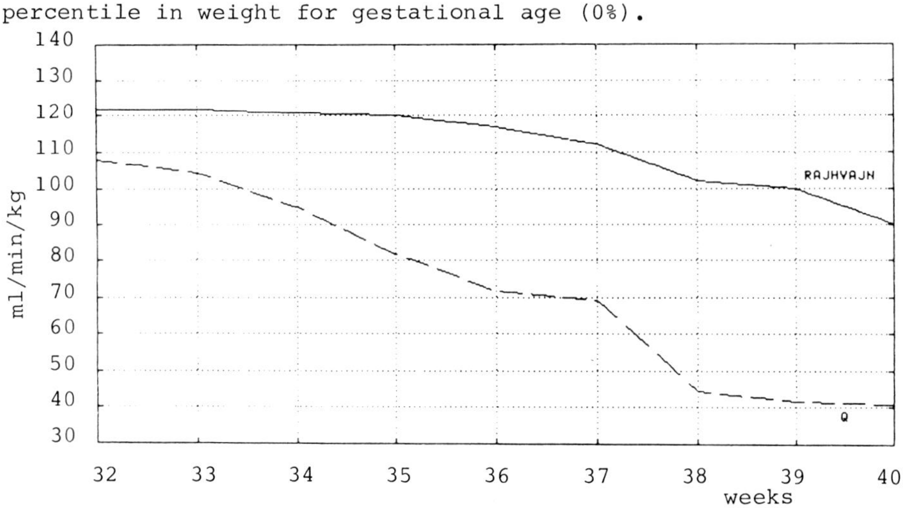

Fig. 5. Fetal umbilical blood flow and hypertonic uterine activity in multigravidas with female infants

In the group with normal uterine activity, birth weight in all fetuses was normal and the outcome was successful. Fetal distress or perinatal death were not observed and all of the babies were delivered vaginally.

In 50 pregnancies where phasic activity was observed two small for dates babies (4,0%) were found but all babies were delivered vaginally in good condition and all survived.

In the third, hypertonic group seven babies (14,0%) had birth weight bellow 5th centile according to Thomson (9). Two out of seven were delivered by Cesarean section with low Apgar score (six or less) and one baby died because of the fetal distress. All seven babies had significantly reduced blood flow values. The average blood flow for all of the small for dates babies was 74,8 ml/min/kg during investigated period. (Table 3.)

TABLE II

INCIDENCE OF SMALL-FOR-DATES BABIES AT BIRTH IN RELATION TO UTERINE ACTIVITY

Uterine activity	Small for dates	Apgar score 6 6	Sectio caesarea	Perinatal mortality
Normal N=100	-	-	-	-
Phasic N=50	2 (4%)	-	-	-
Hypertonic N=50	7 (14%)	2 (4%)	2 (4%)	1 (2%)

DISSCUSSION

Although our hospital has a long experience with electromyography and measurements of uterine activity, the results with EMG and umbilical blood flow were examined during last two years. It is obvious that umbilical blood flow is in the strong correlation with uterine activity, and, in the cases of hypertonus of the uterus, umbilical blood flow is below 2 SD of normal values. Phasic activity does not disturb evidently umbilical blood flow. The incidence of IUGR babies is in the strong corelation with uterine activity and impared utero-placental perfusion. The outcome of pregnancy is in the same corelation. Only in the hypertonic group two babies had fetal distress and were born by Cesarean section, while one baby died. These facts indicate that hypertonic group is, indeed, a high risk group. The duration of monotonous bursts of biopotentials of low amplitude can be prolonged and can even be a characteristic of a particular pregnancy. Classic tocolytic drugs do not have any effect on such a condition because in the majority of cases hypertonus is caused by activation of prostaglandin or histamine receptors. Often tonus does not affect the cervics.

The question is - what is primary and what is secondary process? What is the initial process which will cause the changes of uterine activity and changes in blood flow and lead us to the final result: IUGR fetuses? According to our research uterine activity is one of the basic factors, which can influence and change blood flows. The consequence of reduced feto-maternal circulations are small for date babies.

CONCLUSION

From this investigation, it could be concluded that hypertonic uterine activity occuring in pregnancy can disturb fetal development. Such activity disturbs blood flow in utero-placentary blood vessels. As such pathological activity of myometrium lasts longer, fetal growth retardation occurs. The fetus will be of a lower birth weight, and umbilical vein blood will also be lower. In the case of fetal growth retardation, the state of myometrium should also be absolutely investigated, and reversely, if electromyographically, hypertonic activity of myometrium occurs, the state of fetus should be investigated as well.

REFERENCES

1. Kurjak A, Polak J (1978) J Perinat. Med. Ultrasonic recognition of two types of growth retardation by measurement of four fetal dimension. p 6, 102
2. Rajhvajn B (1982) Beograd, Thesis. Umbilical blood flow measurements in normal and high risk pregnancies
3. Klobučar A (1985) Beograd, Thesis. The influence of pregnant uterine activity on fetal umbilical vein blood flow
4. Eik-Nes SH, Brubakk AO, Ulstein HK (1980) Brit. Med J. 1. Measurements of human fetal blood flow. p 283

5. Leeuwen M (1979) In: Sakamoto SH, Tojo SH, Nakayama I (eds) Uterine contractility. Preceeding of the IX World Congress of gynecology and obstetrics, Tokyo

6. Pronina GM, Zbykovskaya NM (1978) In: Akuŝ. Ginek. The electropulse test - one of the method used in the functional diagnosis at the end pregnancy. pp 7,19

7. Wolfs G, Leeuwen M (1979) In: Acta Obstet. Gynecol. Scand. Suppl. Electromyographyc observations on the human uterus during labor. p 90

8. Kurjak A, Breyer B (1976) In: Amer. J. Obstet. Gynecol. Estimation of Fetal Weight by Ultrasonic Abdominometry. pp 125, 962

9. Thomson A, Billewicz W, Hytten F (1968) In: J. Obstet. Gynae. Br. Cwlth. The assessment of fetal growth. 75:903

UMBILICAL ARTERY BLOOD FLOW VELOCITY WAVEFORMS IN NORMAL AND IUGR FETUSES

ATTILA PÁL and ASIM KURJAK

Ultrasonic Institute, University of Zagreb, "Dr J. Kajfeš" Hospital, Zagreb, Yugoslavia

INTRODUCTION

Among the different methods which examine the placental function, a new method appeard in the last years, the examination of blood flow velocity waveforms of the umbilical artery by ultrasound. These blood flow velocity waveforms were described by McCallum et al. (1) in 1977, but their clinical importance became unquestionable in the last few years. This method enables us to obtain information about the umbilical circulation and about the status of the fetus in a very short period. Disorders occuring to the umbilical circulation during pregnancy and during labour may be grouped into three categories (2): chronic placental disorders, mechanical compromise of the umbilical cord and increase of the vascular resistance of the umbilical circulation. Chronic placental disorders are combined with intrauterine growth retardation of the fetus. The aim of our study was to examine the umbilical artery blood flow velocity waveforms in the asymetrical type of the fetal growth retardation (3) from the 28th week of pregnancy till term, so as to compare these results to the value, which we obtained from eutrophic fetuses.

MATERIAL AND METHOD

The blood flow velocity waveforms of the umbilical artery were examined in 160 healthy pregnant women and 148 intrauterine growth retarded fetuses (IUGR) between the 28th and 41st week of gestation. All healthy pregnant women were free from complaints and they did not use drugs except haemopoetics. None of them was a smoker. In both groups the dates of the last menstrual period were checked for all pregnant women and the lenght of the pregnancy was also confirmed in the last trimester by ultrasound examination in 80 percent of the cases.

The pregnant women average age was 24,2 years in the normal group and 25,2 years in the IUGR group (extreme values in both groups were the same: 17 and 41 years).

All examinations were performed by the same person (A.P.).

Estimation of fetal weight was made using the method described by Kurjak and Breyer (4).

The principle of the examination is based on the Doppler effect: if a static source emits some sound, that is reflecting from a moving surface, the frequency of the sound will change depending on the direction and the velocity of the moving object. If the direction of the moving object is near the receiver, the frequency increases, if it is departing from the receiver the frequency decreases. The frequency change is in direct proportion with the velocity of the moving object. These frequency changes are called Doppler shift. If the ultrasound beam moves towards a vessel the moving erythrocytes function as reflecting surface and they change the frequency of the reflected ultrasound. Doppler shift can be described according to the following equation.

$$f_d = \frac{2 \times f_o \times \bar{v} \times \cos \Theta}{c}$$

f_d = Doppler shift

f_o = frequency of the emitted sound

v = velocity of the reflecting surface

Θ = angle between the direction of the ultrasound beam and the moving, reflecting object

c = velocity of the ultrasound in the examined material (in blood 1570 m/sec)

Doppler shift is audible to human ears, provided that the frequency of the emitted sound is between 1-lo MHz. Hence, the changes of the velocity, or the velocity itself can be made audible.

A Kranzbühler 8130 Duplex Doppler machine was used in all examinations. The linear transducer (3 MHz) was connected with the Doppler transducer (2 MHz) in 50°. The direction of the Doppler ultrasound beam and the sample volume were controlled on the monitor. The frequency analysis was performed by a computer built in machine using the Discrete Fourier Transformation.

The examination was performed as follows: the position of the fetus was located by means of the linear transducer. The circumference of the abdomen was measured at the height of umbilical vein and fetal weight was estimated on the basis of this result (4).

The biparietal diameter was measured, as well. Then the umbilical cord was searched by means of linear transducer. In most cases it was located without difficulty, as it can be seen at the opposite side of the fetus or between the fetal extremities. Subsequently the Doppler ultrasound beam was directed to the umbilical loop and the sample volume was set.The typical sound and sign of the umbilical artery is shown on the monitor. Sometimes (e.g. oligohydramnion) it was not possible to visualize the umbilical branch. In these cases we searched at the above mentioned places with the Doppler ultrasound beam and the typical aound signal and the waveform made the waveform analysis possible in all of the cases.

The studies made during periods of fetal activity or breathing movements were not used, e.g. when there is active fetal breathing, there is a sinus arrhytmia , which makes measurement of ratios difficult because the altering pulse intervals result in different diastolic levels. A typical example can be seen in Figure 1.

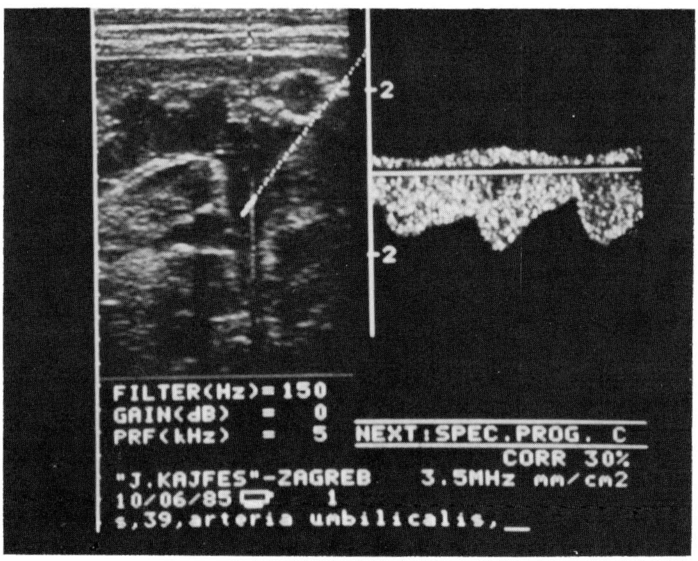

The left side of the Polaroid picture illustrates the uterine wall, fetal extremities, fetal body and the umbilical branch. The dotted line images the direction of the Doppler beam and the bright up area is the time gate. The right side of the ultrasonogram shows the velocity waveforms of the umbilical artery (lower channel). During the examination there was a continuous fetal breathing movement.

All shapes of the pulse waves are different, which indicates a changing stream in the umbilical vessels in every cardiac cycle.

Evaluation of the values was made using A/B ratio (5), Resistance Index ($RI = \frac{A - B}{A}$) (6), where A = systolic peak, B = end diastole.

For statistical analysis the Student - t test and hi-square test were used.

RESULTS

Between the 28th and 39th week of pregnancy there was a significantly lower estimated fetal weight ($p < 0{,}001$) in the IUGR group than in the normal group (Fig. 2).

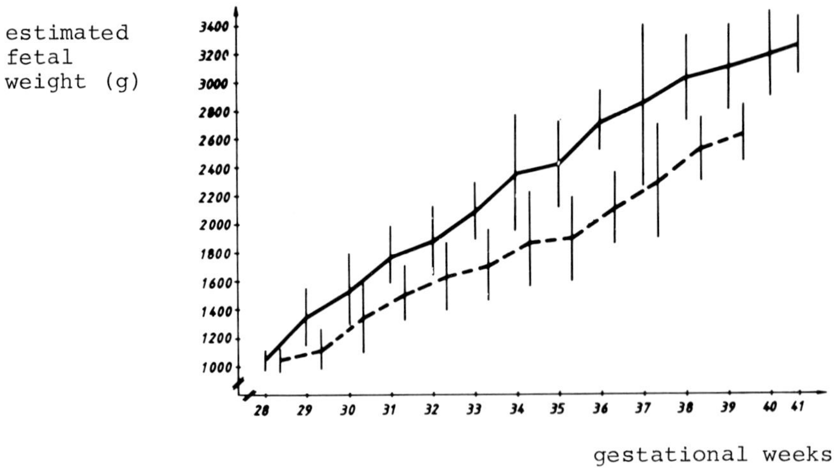

———	n= 5	11	12	12	9	lo	13	14	15	12	13	13	11	10
												(normal)		
----	n= 8	7	9	14	lo	lo	14	13	19	15	lo	19	-	-
												(IUGR)		

Changes of the estimated fetal weight in eutrophic and IUGR fetuses during the third trimester of pregnancy.

In Figure 3 we present the change of the A/B ratios and Resistance Indexes. In normal pregnancy the A/B ratio decreases from 3,0 - 2,5 to 2,0 or less and the Resistance Index from 0,6 to 0,5 during the third trimester. The decreasing tendency was continuous.

A/B

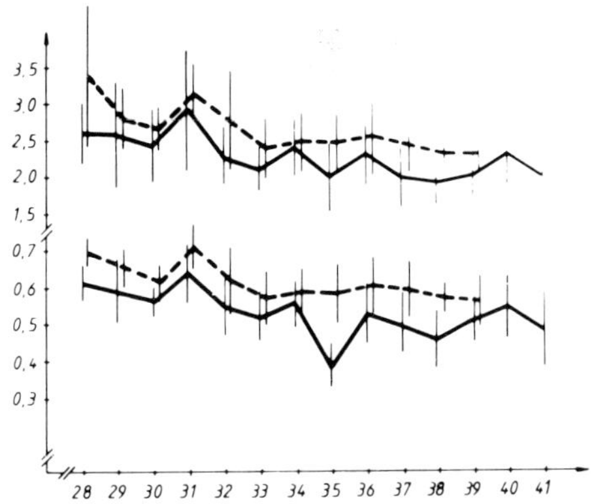

RI

gestational weeks

n= 5 11 12 12 9 lo 13 14 15 16 13 13 11 lo

(normal)

n= 8 7 9 14 lo lo 14 13 19 15 lo 19 - -

(IUGR)

Change of the A/B ratio (A= systolic peak, B= end diastole) and Resistance Index (RI $= \frac{A - B}{A}$) in the umbilical artery during the third trimester of pregnancy.

In IUGR fetuses the A/B ratio decreases from 3,5 - 3,0 to 2,5 and the Resistance Index from 0,7 to 0,6. The most drastic difference between the two curves was that the decreasing tendency in IUGR fetuses stopped at about the 33rd week of pregnancy. From this time the A/B ratio as well as the Resistance Index were near by the same level in IUGR fetuses and showed a higher resistance of vascular placental bed than in normal pregnancies.

The velocity waveforms were continuously above the zero line (Fig. 4) in normal pregnancies. This fact shows a continuous forward flow, during the diastole. If the velocity waveforms return to the zero line it indicates no forward flow during diastole for a short period (Fig. 5). This case was an IUGR fetus in middle degree: comparing Figure 5 with Figure 6, which was made on the same gestational week, one can see the difference in diastolic flow. Comparing Figure 4 to Figure 6, one can see how during the third trimester in normal case, the diastolic flow become stronger.

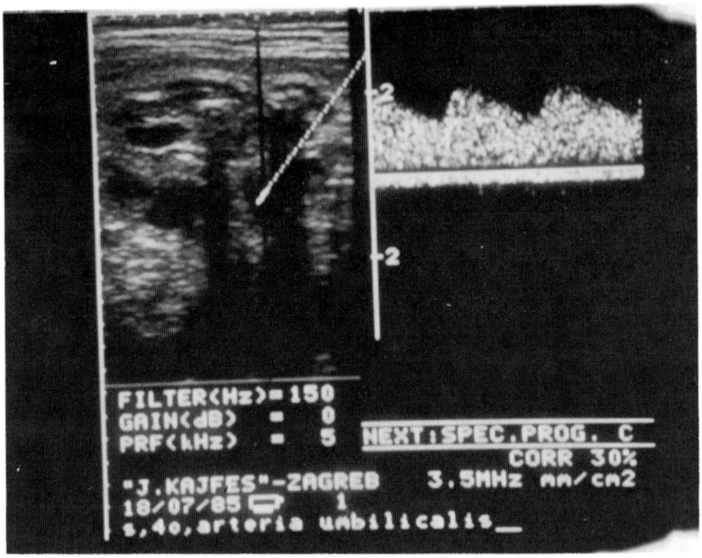

Fig. 4. The sonogram displays the umbilical artery velocity waveforms on the 40th week of a normal pregnancy. The direction of the Doppler ultrasound beam is indicated by the dotted line and at its end, the traced line shows the time gate (left side of the picture). The typical velocity waveforms of the umbilical artery can be seen on the upper channel (right side of the picture). In normal pregnancy, the blood flow has a high systolic and high diastolic velocity in the umbilical artery.

Fig. 5. Umbilical artery velocity waveforms on the 29th week of pregnancy in a IUGR fetus. In the whole cardiac cycle the waveforms fall to the zero line during diastole, indicating an absence of the forward flow for a short period.

Figure 6. Umbilical artery velocity waveforms on the 29th week of pregnancy in a normal fetus. During the diastole the waveforms are continuously above the zero line, indicating a persistent forward flow.

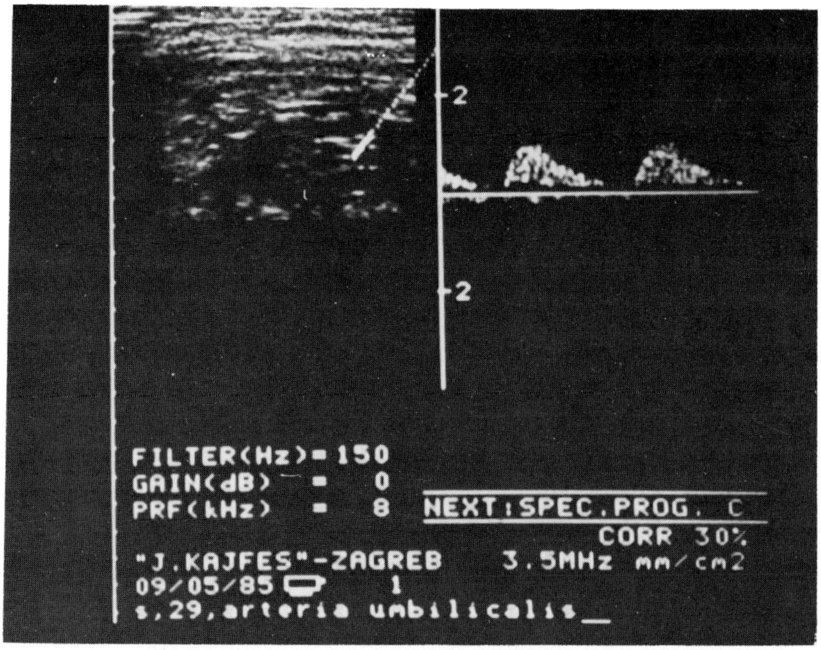

Figure 5

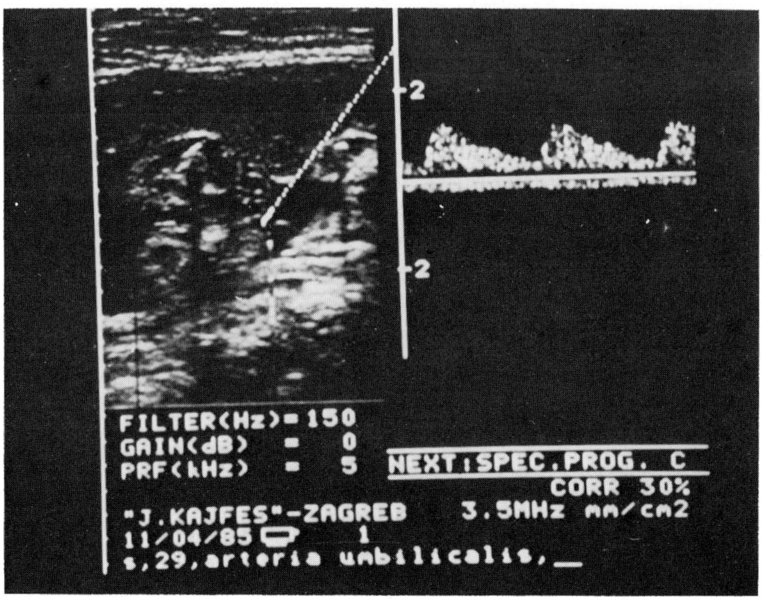

Figure 6

A very severe IUGR case is shown in Figure 7. The velocity waveforms always fall down to the zero line at the end of

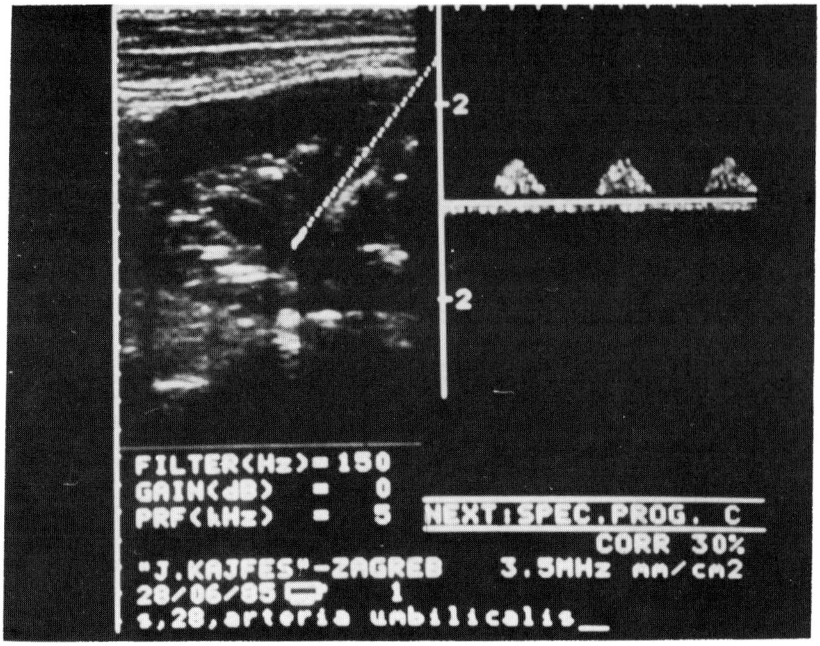

Figure 7. Umbilical artery velocity waveforms in the 28th week of pregnancy in a very severe IUGR fetus. After systole, the velocity waveforms fall immediately to the zero line. This case represents an absolute absence of umbilical artery circulation during the whole diastole.

systole. This indicates that there is no blood circulation in the umbilical artery during the whole period of diastole. This fetus died in utero 12 days after the examination.

In Table I we summerised the results of the examninations of umbilical artery blood flow velocity waveforms, and compared with the fifth minute Apgar score. The result of the waveform analysis was regarded as a pathological value (according to our own normal curve), if the A/B ratio was higher than 3,0 and/or the RI was higher than 0,66. In all of the cases the Apgar score was determined in the first and fifth minute of life, but for evaluation of the results we used only the fifth minute Apgar score. From Table I the following basic conclusions can be made. There are significantly more:

- normal waveforms than pathological one in eutrophic fetuses ($p < 0,01$)
- the high Apgar points (lo-7) than the low Apgar points (< 7) in eutrophic fetuses with normal waveforms ($p < 0,01$)
- the low Apgar points (< 7) in eutrophic fetuses with pathological waveforms than with normal one ($p < 0,01$)
- the high Apgar points (lo-7) in IUGR fetuses with normal waveforms ($p < 0,01$)
- the high Apgar points (lo-7) in IUGR fetuses with normal waveforms than the low Apgar points ($p < 0,01$)
- the low Apgar points (< 7) in IUGR fetuses with pathological waveforms than the high Apgar points ($p < 0,01$)
- the low Apgar points (< 7) at IUGR fetuses with pathological waveforms than with normal waveforms ($p < 0,01$)
- the pathological waveforms at IUGR fetuses than eutrophic ones ($p < 0,01$)
- the low Apgar points (< 7) at IUGR fetuses with normal waveforms than at eutrophic fetuses with normal waveforms ($p < 0,01$)

TABLE I

Apgar score 5th min.	Eutrophic fetuses (n=160)		IUGR fetuses (n=148)	
	Normal (n=156)	Pathological (n=4)	Normal (n=128)	Pathological (n=20)
	Waveforms		Waveforms	
10-7	148	1	100	4
6-4	6	3	22	12
3-0	2	0	6	4

Table I. Correlation between the result of the examination of the umbilical artery velocity waveforms in eutrophic and IUGR fetuses and the status of the newborn.

The intra-observer failure examination took place as follows. Measurements were repeated every ten minutes in the same pregnant woman by the same examinatior. A total of 10 pregnant women was examined this way. No significant difference could be found ($p > 0,05$) when comparing both groups concerning the A/B ratio and Resistance Index.

DISCUSSION

Beside the fetal cardiac force and the status of the blood vessel walls the resistance of the placental bed is another factor determining blood flow in the umbilical aetery. Depending on the degree of this resistance, the blood is reflected at different degree in the umbilical artery. If the resistance of the placental bed is low, the reflection is also low, thus there is continuous forward flow during the diastole. The low A/B ratio and the low Resistance Index show this continuous, strong, forward flow during diastole.

In normal pregnancy both the A/B ratio and Resistance Index show a continuous decreasing tendency during the third trimester. Our result is similar to the result obtained by Trudinger et al. (7), Stuart et al. (5) and Schuman et al. (8). This statement supports the idea that the vessel resistance of the placental bed continuously decreases during the third trimester of the pregnancy.

A possible cause of these changes is the increase in the number of tertiary stem villi during the third trimester as well. Another cause may be, that the trophoblast is rich in prostaglandins, thus causing a local vasodilatation.

According to Trudinger et al. (9) fetuses with an abnormal umbilical study were delivered earlier ($p < 0,01$) and were more likely to reuire neonatal intensive care admission ($p < 0,001$). This statement was also supported by our results. As all our figures indicate after the 39th week of pregnancy, the results of IUGR fetuses, were not calculated, due to a small number of patients, preventing a statistical comparison of the groups.

Schulman et al. (8) examined 89 eutrophic fetuses between the 25th and 42nd week of pregnsncy 162 times and 15 IUGR fetuses from 29th to 40th gestational week 40 times. It was found that the A/B ratio decreased from 2,8 to 2,2 in normal fetuses and decreased from 3,8 to 3,0 in IUGR fetuses during the examnined period.

Fleisher et al. (11) examined 189 pregnant women 587 times between the 18th and 42nd week of pregnancy. They defined the A/B as abnormal if ≥ 3. In IUGR fetuses the test was positive in 32 cases and negative in 7 cases. In eutrophic fetuses the test was positive in 26 cases and negative in 124 cases. It was found that the A/B ratio is significantly higher at IUGR fetuses than at eutrophic fetuses.

Trudinger et al. (7) examined 43 IUGR fetuses. They found reduced, absent or reverse flow during the diastole in 32 cases. In all fetuses the result of the A/B ratio was in the normal range (3,1 - 2,4 the 50th percent from 28th to 40th week of gestation). In another study the same group (9) examined 88 suspected IUGR fetuses. 62 abnormal umbilical artery blood flow velocity waveforms were found. Of the 62 fetuses 39 had "bad" and 23 had "good" fetal outcome.

Giles et al. (11) examined the umbilical artery blood flow velocity waveforms in 76 twin pregnancies. From these pregnancies, 33 had one or both fetuses IUGR. Among these IUGR fetuses in 78 percent (20) had elevated A/B ratio.

Summarizing and comparing the literature with our results the following conclusions can be drown:

- the examination of the umbilical artery blood flow velocity waveforms is a very good and quick method to get information about fetal status in utero. If a pathological waveform at one eutrophic fetus is obtained other examinations, are also necessary (e.g. cardiotocography, examination of the oestriol, HPL etc.), to get more precise information about the fetus condition. If we get a pathological waveform at an IUGR fetus the termination of the pregnancy is to be considered. This practical conclusion may bring useful and new benefits in the field of perinatology.

CONCLUSION

Blood flow velocity waveform of the umbilical artey were examined in 160 healthy pregnant women and 148 intrauterine growth retarded fetuses (IUGR) between the 28th and 41st week of gestation. A Kranzbühler 8130 Duplex Doppler machine was used in all examinations.

Evaluation of the results was performed using A/B ratios and Resistance Indexes ($RI = \frac{A - B}{A}$), where A= systolic peak, B= end diastole.

In norml pregnancy the A/B ratio decreases from 3,0-2,5 to 2,0 or less, and the Resistance Index from 0.7 to 0.6. The decreasing tendency was continuous. In IUGR fetuses the A/B ratio decreases from 3.5 - 3.0 to 2.5 and the Resistance Index from 0.7 to 0.6. The decreasing tendency of the curve in IUGR fetuses ceased at about the 33rd week of pregnancy and remained at the same level.

There were significantly more pathological waveforms in IUGR fetuses than in eutrophic ones ($p > 0.01$).

REFERENCES

1. McCallum WD, Olson RF, Daigle PE, Baker DW (1977) Real-time analysis of Doppler signals obtained by the feto-placental circulation. In: White D and Brown KE (eds) Ultrasound in Medicine, New York, Plenum Publishing Corp.
2. Künzel W (1981) Umbilical circulation - physiology and pathology. J. of Perinatal Medicine. Supp. 1 9:68-71
3. Kurjak A, Beazley JM, Latin V, Funduk-Kurjak B (1980) Fetal growth retardation and EPH gestosis In: Current status of EPH gestosis. Kurjak A, Rippmann T, Sulovič V (eds) Excerpta Medica, Amsterdam-Oxford-Princeton, pp 340-352
4. Kurjak A, Breyer B. Estimation of fetal weight by ultrasonic abdominometry. Amer. J. Obstet. Gynecol. 125:962,1976
5. Stuart D, Drumm J, Fitzgerald DL, Duigan NM (1980) Fetal blood velocity waveforms in normal pregnancy. Brit. J. Obstet. Gynaecol. 87:780-785
6. Pourcelot L (1974) Applications cliniques de l'examen Doppler trancutanie. In: Peronneau P: In velocimetric ultrasonor Doppler 34:625
7. Trudinger BJ, Giles WB, Cook CM, Bombardieri J, Collins L (1985) Fetal umbilical artery flow velocity waveforms and placental resistance: clinical significance. Brit. J. Obstet. Gynecol. 92:23-30
8. Schulman H, Fleischer A, Stern W, Farmakides G, Jagani N, Blattner P (1984) Umbilical velocity wave ratios in human pregnancy. Amer. J. Obstet. Gynecol. 148:985-990
9. Trudinger BJ, Giles WB, Cook CM (1985) Flow velocity waveforms in the maternal uteroplacental and fetal umbilical placental circulations. Am. J. Obstet. Gynecol. 152:155-163
10. Fleisher A, Schulman H, Farmakides G, Bracero L, Blattner P, Randolf G (1985) Umbilical artery velocity waveforms and intrauterine growth retardation. Am. J. Obstet. Gynecol. 151: 502-505
11. Giles WB, Trudinger BJ, Cook CM (1985) Fetal umbilical artery flow velocity-time waveforms in twin pregnancies. Br. J. Obstet. Gynecol. 92:490-497

STUDIES ON PULSED ULTRASONIC FLOW METRY, ULTRASONIC COLOR DOPPLER TECHNIQUE AND THE EVALUATION OF CONTINUOUS WAVE ULTRASONIC DOPPLER FLOW METRY

K. MAEDA, K. ISHIHARA and Y. TAKEUCHI

Department of Obstetrics and Gynecology, Tottori University School of Medicine, Yonago 683 Japan

INTRODUCTION

The clinical value of blood flow measurement was evaluated in conventional pulsed ultrasonic Doppler flow metry, the experience of so-called color Doppler method and the newly introduced continuous wave (CW) ultrasonic Doppler method. Some other techniques of fetal diagnosis were used with the flow metry including fetal heart rate (FHR) monitoring and the fetal actogram (Maeda, 1985).

PULSED ULTRASONIC DOPPLER FLOW STUDIES IN EPH-GESTOSIS

The conventional blood flow metry analyzed with FFT has been studied with use of pulsed Doppler device in maternal iliac artery that was mainly external one, and also in umbilical cord artery of the fetus. The initial parameter was blood flow volume, and the most remarkable finding was its change in maternal iliac artery after postural change. Maternal iliac arterial flow volume increased by the change to lateral recumbent position on the other side from supine posture.

Since Campbell et al (1985) reported the importance of blood flow profile and the wave form analyis in the mother and fetus, the pulsatility index of the iliac arterial blood flow and the resistance index of fetal arterial flow were investigated in the present report. The pulsatility index of maternal iliac arterial flow increased significantly in the gestosis cases who showed hypertension and/or proteinuria when compared to normal pregnancy. However, the change was insignificant in the cases who showed simple edema (Fig. 1). The peripheral vascular resistance would be larger in the cases of severe EPH-gestosis than normal pregnancy.

Similar finding was noted in the resistance index of umbilical arterial blood flow, namely, the resistance index was significantly higher in the gestosis cases with hypertension and/or proteinuria than normal pregnancy, though the index did not increase in the gestosis cases with simple edema. From the results, it was postulated that the resistance of fetal peripheral artery increased in the cases of severe EPH-gestosis (Fig. 2).

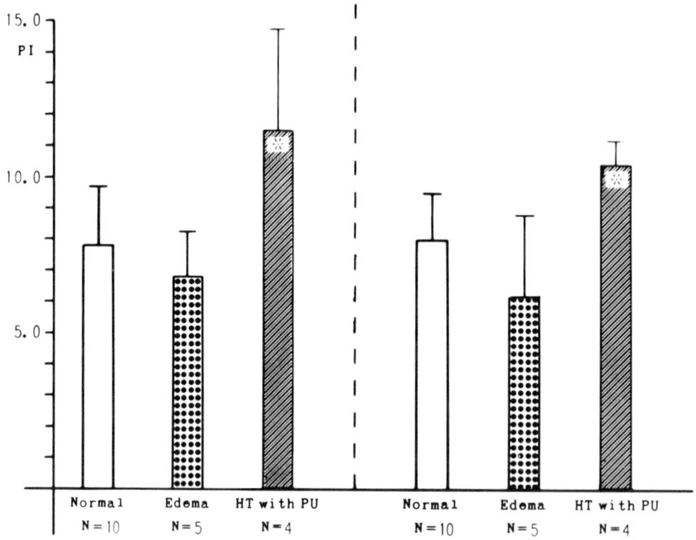

Fig. 1. The pulsatility index values obtained in left (left figure) and right (right figure) iliac arteries of EPH-gestosis cases. White bars show the values of normal pregnancy, grey bars gestosis with simple edema, and black bars the values of gestosis with hypertension and/or proteinuria. The index showed significant increase in the cases of gestosis with hypertension and/or proteinuria.

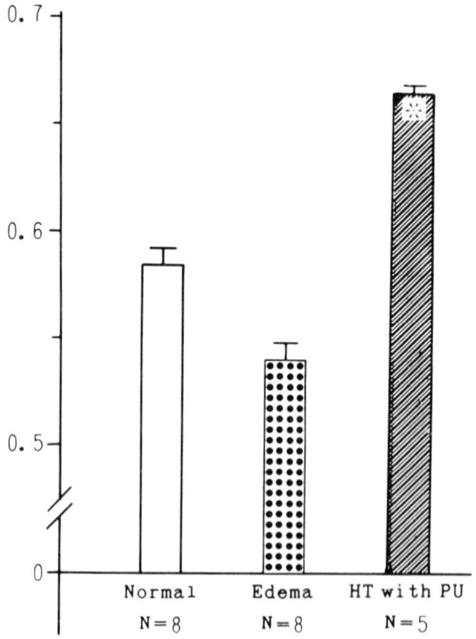

Fig. 2. The resistance index of umbilical cord arterial blood flow increased in the cases of severe EPH-gestosis with hypertension and/or proteinuria (black bar) when compared to normal pregnancy (white bar), while the simple edema case showed significant decrease of the index (grey bar).

THE COLOR DOPPLER TECHNIQUE STUDIED ON FETAL CIRCULATION

Method

Recently, the blood flow is determined by a new color Doppler method which is the color display of blood flow on ultrasonic B-mode image. The new technique has been mainly used in the cardiac blood flow of adult patient, since simultaneous display of verious kinds of blood flow with several directions was needed in the realization of intracardiac blood flow. Aloka 880 ultrasonograph has been used in the diagnosis of adult heart disease in our university hospital.

The part where blood flow is present is displayed by red or blue color on the B-mode screen. Red means the existence of forward flow at the part, and blue away flow. The color brightness is divided into 4 grades, dark to light according to flow velocity which is determined by the Doppler frequency detected with autocorrelation technique. Therefore, the blood vessels are easily recognized on the screen with the method. The flow velocity is not very quantatively displayed, since the color brightness has only 4 grades. However, further advantage of the method is the detection of the variance of flow velocity in a vessel, and the phenomenon is displayed by the mixing of green color.

Materials and Results

The color Doppler method was tried in the recognition of fetal blood flow in fetal body during pregnancy. Intracardiac flow was clear in the four chamber view of the fetal B-mode display. The outflow into the aorta was also clearly shown, and the variance of blood flow was detected by mixing green color. Fetal blood flow was noted in various vessels easily, and umbilical cord artery and vein were displayed with different colors, and the discrimination was possble between the artery and vein with the method. Systolic and diastolic blood flow were also displayed with red and blue colors alternatively on M-mode record of fetal cardiac ventricular contraction with the technique (Fig. 3).

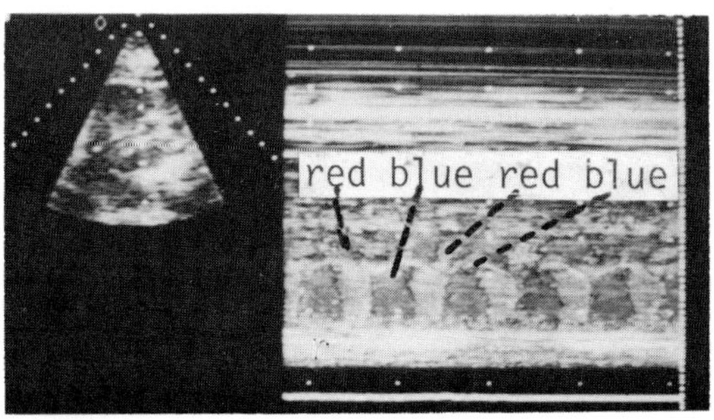

Fig. 3. Color Doppler displays on B-mode (left) and M-mode (right) of fetal heart with Aloka 880. Intracardiac flow is shown by red color in the B-mode. Systole is displayed by red and diastole by blue alternatively in the M-mode.

From these experiences, it is postulated that the blood vessels will be easily detected in fetal body, and abnormal blood flow will be rapidly recognized in the structural abnormality of fetal heart or in the large vessel anomaly.

CONTINUOUS WAVE ULTRASONIC DOPPLER FLOW METRY

Methods and Materials

Recently, the importance of blood flow profile, the wave form, the level of diastole in the profile, the ratio of systole to the end-diastole, the resistance index or pulsatility index is reported in the study of fetal great vessel and maternal arquate artery in the pregnancy. All of the reports have described the determination of frequency ratio in the wave form, but not discussed the absolute value. The ratio of systolic frequency to that of end-diastole is possibly determined by CW ultrasonic Doppler method in the blood flow profile which does not include the reverse flow but the pulsating wave is superimposed on continuous flow pattern. Such blood flow as described above has been reported in fetal great vessels, fetal aorta, umbilical artery and in maternal arquate artery. Hence, it was considered not meaningless to investigate the CW ultrasonic Doppler technique in blood flow metry, if the use is limited in suitable blood flow. The equipment suitable to the purpose was reported by Maeda (1969) which was composed of conventional CW ultrasonic fetal heart detector, frequency demodulator and a recorder. Fetal arterial blood flow in the placenta was clearly recorded in the report with use of the simple device.

An ultrasonic Doppler fetal heart detector of which CW ultrasound frequency was 2MHz, frequency demodulator composed of Schmitt trigger, monostable multivibrator of which pulse duration was 0.22ms and RC circuit integrator with the time constant of 0.03sec, and a heat-pen recorder were used in this study.

Initial subjects were own carotid artery, femoral artery and various small arteries of the first author. After realizing the characteristics of the device, 6 cases of normal and abnormal pregnant cases were investigated with the CW flow metry device.

Results

Adult subjects. The carotid blood flow showed the variation accoding to the distance from the heart in the own trials for the investigator's arteries. The flow curve of femoral artery disappeared after compression of central part, and reappeared after the decompression. Small arteries are also clearly detected in ophthalmic artery in the orbita, facial artery located under the chin and the palmar branch of radial artery (Fig. 4). The sensitivity and discriminating ability of flow pattern were postulated to be sufficient from these experiences.

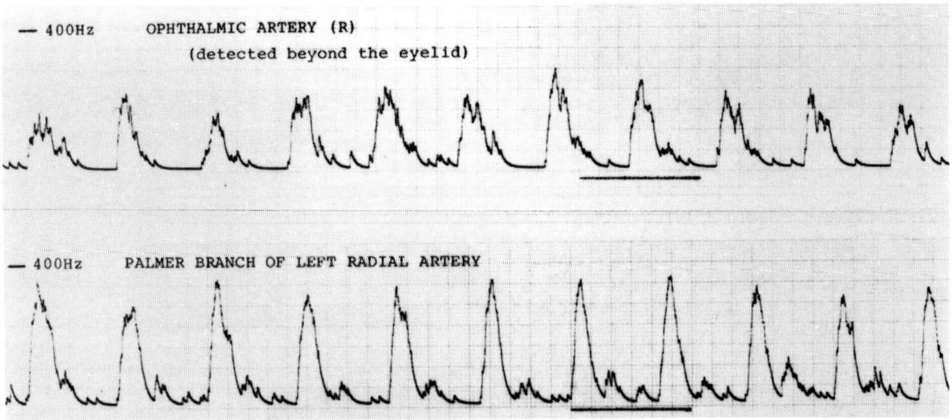

Fig. 4. CW ultrasonic Doppler blood flow curves of a male adult. Upper; right ophthalmic artery in the orbita. Lower; palmar branch of left radial artery.

Results obtained in pregnant cases.

Case 1. 34 weeks of pregnancy, EPH-gestosis, non-reactive NST. The CW ultrasonic method was compared to the conventional pulsed Ultrasonic Doppler flow metry in the case. Maternal right external iliac artery flow pattern obtained by pulsed Doppler method showed a typical external iliac pattern which combined the reverse flow. In the same artery, the CW flow metry showed no reverse flow part in spite of clear similarity of the wave form in forward flow. Peak frequency in the pulsed method was 1,600Hz, and that of CW method was approximately 600Hz. Since the CW method shows average frequency, the value will baout 2/3 of the instantaneous peak value of the pulsed method. In addition the ultrasound frequency was 3.5MHz in pulsed method, and the CW ultrasound 2MHz. Hence, the peak systolic frequency of the CW method will be about 2/3 x 2/3.5 of the pulsed one. It will be about 600Hz if 1,600Hz is multiplied by the factor. Therefore, the frequency similarity is obtained between these two methods (Fig. 5).

Umbilical artery was detected by B-mode and the CW method was applied on the artery. The conventional pulsed Doppler method was compared with the CW. No reverse flow was noted in the artery, and the two patterns obtained by pulsed and CW methods are similar in the wave form. Peak frequency of pulsed method was about 1,000Hz, and it will be about 400Hz if the factor is multiplied. Actual value of the CW method was about 500Hz, and not very much different from the calculated value. The ratio of systole/end-diastole frequencies was 2.7 in the pulsed Doppler flow pattern, and 3.4 in CW method. These differences between pulsed Doppler and CW method will be explained by unstable location of umbilical cord which was floated in amniotic fluid (Fig. 5)

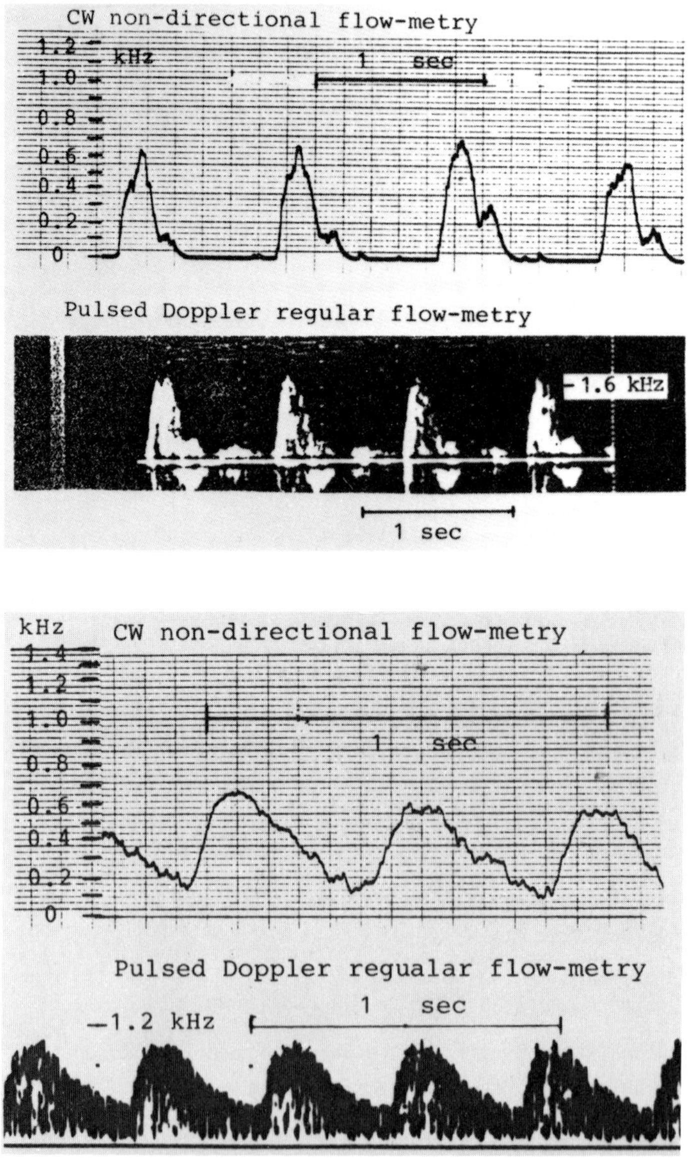

Fig. 5. Comparison of the wave forms obtained by CW ultrasonic Doppler method and the pulsed ultrasonic Doppler. Upper figure was obtained at maternal external iliac artery. The lower one was recorded in ubilical cord artery. Upper curves are the CW method, and lower ones pulsed ultrasonic Doppler method.

Case 2. 40 weeks, normal pregnancy. External iliac artery was very clear, but internal iliac was hardly identified and suspected by the wave form and the location of artery. Systole/diastole ratio was 2.4 in suspected internal iliac. Fetal aortic flow was hardly separated from fetal heart signal in the listening to Doppler sound, though the curve was recorded. However, fetal artery located in the placenta was clear from its fixed location, beating rate and pulsating nature of the sound. Systole/diastole ratio was 1.6 in the placental arterial flow pattern (Fig. 6).

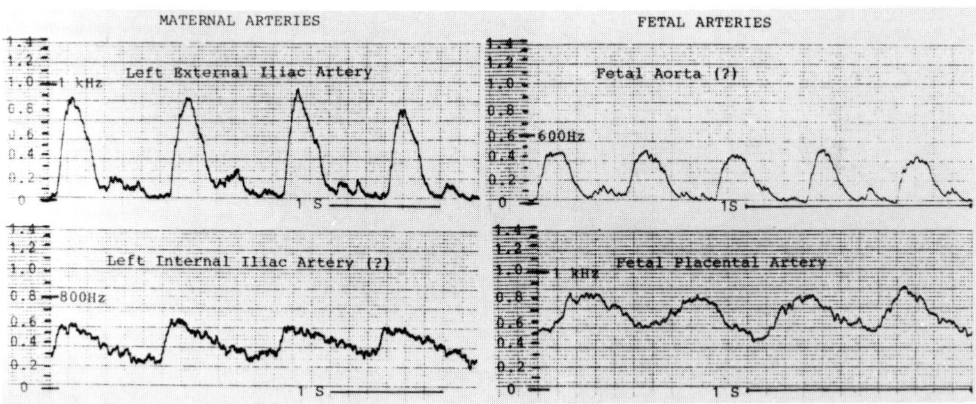

Fig. 6. Maternal and fetal arterial flow patterns in Case 2. Left half shows external iliac artery (upper) and suspected internal iliac (lower). Right half is the fetal flow profiles, and upper is suspected fetal aorta which was hardly separated from fetal heart signal. Right lower is fetal artery located in the placenta, and high end-diastolic frequency is characteristic.

Case 3. 20 weeks and complicated with large uterine fibromyoma. Maternal flow was recorded in bilateral external iliac, femoral and suspected internal iliac arteries. In spite of combined large fibromyoma and early stage of pregnancy, the flow in fetal large vessel, suspectedly fetal aorta, was recorded (Fig. 7).

Case 4. 28 weeks, left nephrectomized. No obstetric complication. Bilateral external iliac arteries were clearly recorded by the CW method, but the internal or uterine artery was hardly identified. Flow profile of aorta or large vessel of the fetus was recorded, and systole/diastole ratio was about 2 in the case. Placental vein flow was recorded by CW method, though it was hardly identified (Fig. 8).

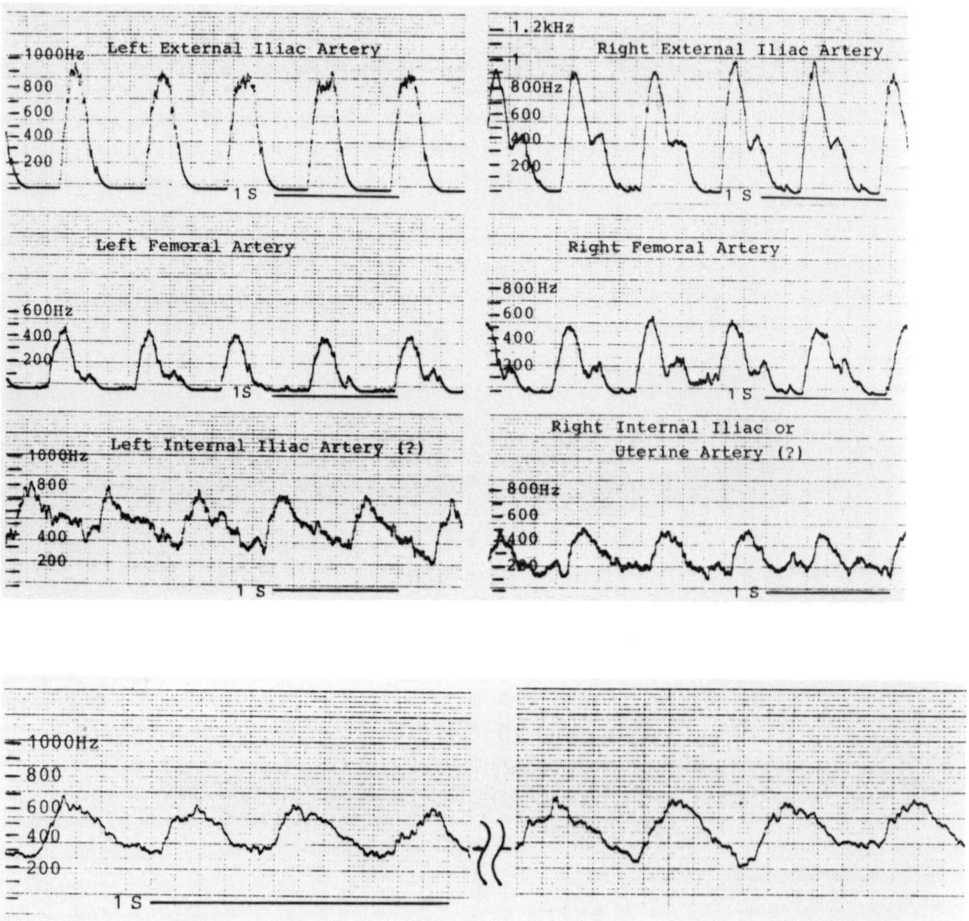

(A)

(B)

Fig. 7. Case 3. 20 weeks and uterine fibromyoma. (A) shows bilateral external iliac (upper), femoral (middle) and suspected internal iliac (lower) arteries. (B) was obtained in large fetal artery.

Case 5. 28 weeks, normal pregnancy. Bilateral external iliac and left suspected internal iliac artery flow profiles were clearly recorded, while right internal iliac was vague. Fetal large vessel profile was suspected to be aorta, and placental fetal artery was clearly identified and recorded (Fig. 9).

Case 6. 34 weeks, EPH-gestosis, IUGR, non-reactive NST and also no reaction to fetal movement on fetal actogram, mild FHR deceleration, and the loss of acceleration. Chronic fetal hypoxia was suspected from these changes. External iliac artery was clearly recorded, but insufficiently in internal. Fetal placen-

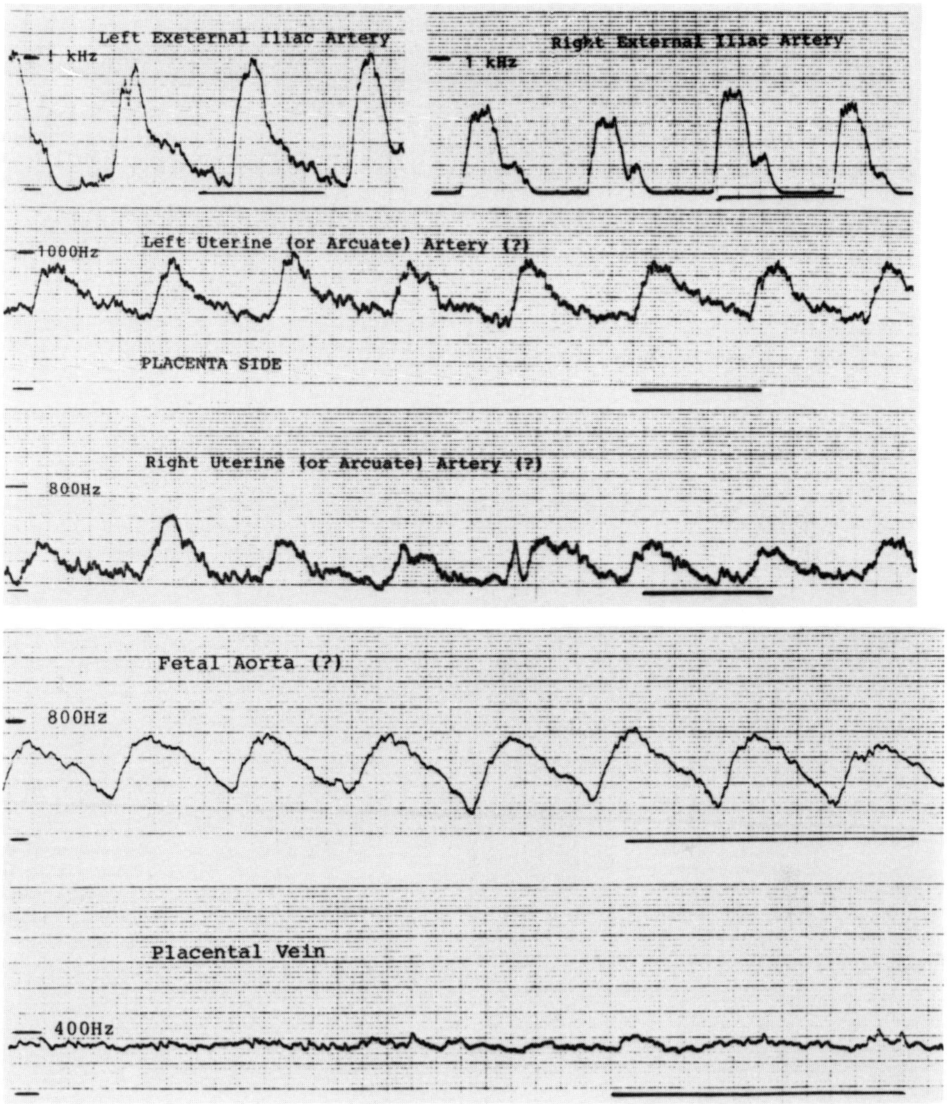

(A)

(B)

Fig. 8. Case 4. 20 weeks, left nephrectomized. (A) upper shows bilateral iliac artery profiles, the middle left uterine arquate artery suspected, the lower of that right side. (B) is fetal aortic or large artery flow, and the lower placental vein flow.

tal artery was clearly recorded. The flow profile of umbilical cord artery, that was confirmed by B-mode, showed low end-diastole, and systole/diastole ratio was as high as 7.5 in the state of fetal normocardia. The intervals of systole peaks was elongated at FHR deceleration which was confirmed on FHR chart, and the FHR calculated from the flow profile dropped to 92bpm at the deceleration from 125bpm at the state of normocardia. Systolic peak frequency was 500Hz at fetal normocardia, and 650Hz in FHR deceleration. The frequency increased as the heart rate decreased, namely, flow velocity increased at the deceleration. This means the increase of fetal cardiac output at decreased heart rate. The mechanism was also estimated by elongated duration of every flow curve at the deceleration. The recording was done urgently at the bed side, and cesarean section was carried out after the test, since fetal distress was diagnosed in the patient.

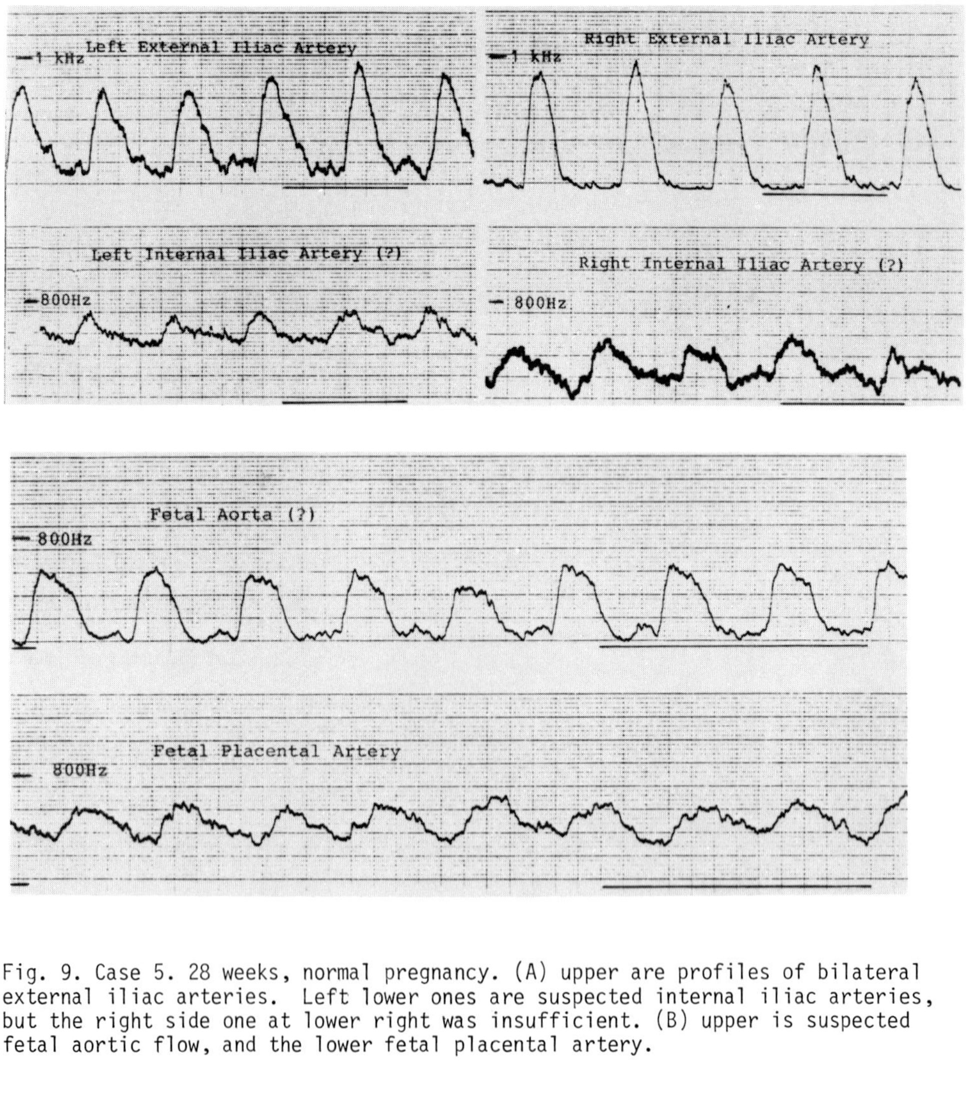

Fig. 9. Case 5. 28 weeks, normal pregnancy. (A) upper are profiles of bilateral external iliac arteries. Left lower ones are suspected internal iliac arteries, but the right side one at lower right was insufficient. (B) upper is suspected fetal aortic flow, and the lower fetal placental artery.

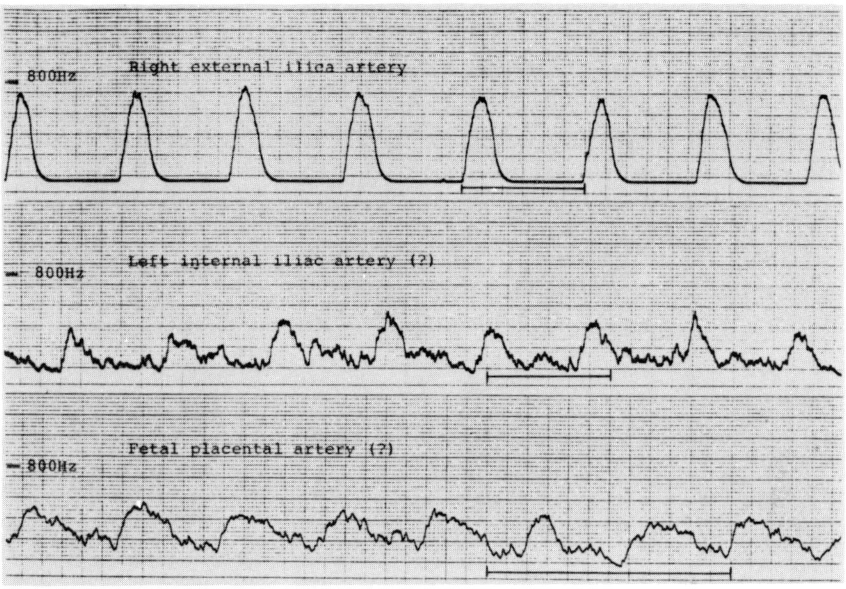

(A)

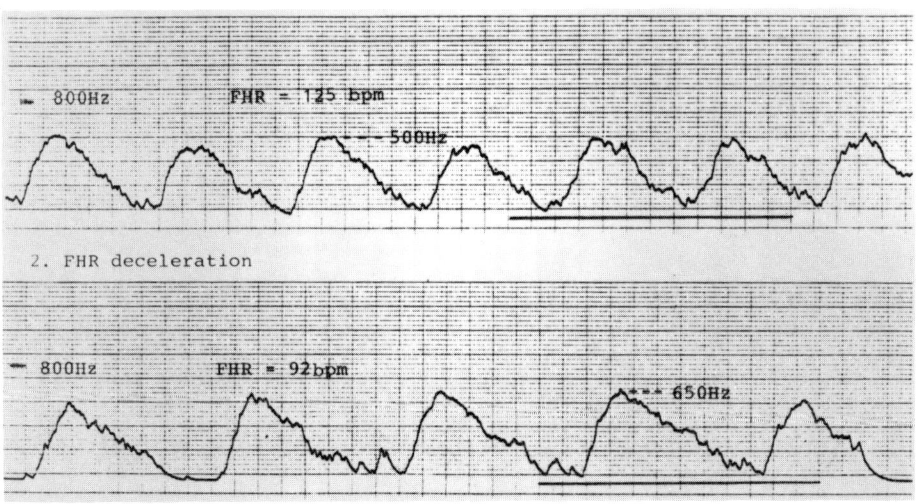

(B)

Fig. 10. Case 6. 34 weeks, IUGR, chronic fetal hypoxia, cesarea section. (A) upper curves are recorded at external and suspected internal iliac arteries. Lower one is fetal placental artery. (B) upper flow profile was obtained at umbilical cord artery at normocardia. Lower was recorded at FHR deceleration. Increased peak frequency at 650 Hz from 500 and elongated wave form suggest increased fetal cariac output at FHR deceleration.

Conclusion

Peak-averaged blood flow profile was recorded by nondirectional CW ultrasonic Doppler method. 1) Ultrasonic Doppler frequency was comparable in the methods of pulsed Doppler and the CW Doppler. 2) External iliac artery was clearly identified with CW method. Internal iliac or uterine artery was supposedly identified by its location, Doppler sound and wave form. Large arterial flow in fetal body was clearly recorded,though the identification was not easy in CW method. Fetal artery in the placenta was easily identified. 3) Systole/diastole frequency ratio of umbilical arterial flow was high in a fetus of IUGR and hypoxia in the CW method. Systolic frequency increased at FHR deceleration suggesting fetal cardiac output increase in fetal bradycardia. 6) The CW device was small, easy to handle, monitored by Doppler sound, and utilized at bed side even in emergency case.

REFERENCES

1. Campbell S. Cohen-Overbeek T (1985) Clinical value of blood-flow measurement in pregnancy. In Kurjak A(ed) The Fetus as a Patient. Excerpta Medica, Amsterdam, pp 300-311

2. Maeda K, Kimura S, Fukui Y, Ozawa S, Kosaka T, Wang C, Tamura M, Takata D, Nakano H, Mitoma M (1969) Pathophysiology of Fetus, Fukuoka Printing

3. Maeda K, Tatsumura T, Takeuchi K, Oota M, Minagawa Y, Irie T (1985) Modern technology and the fetus. In Kurjak A(ed) The Fetus as a Patient. Excerpta Medica, Amsterdam, pp 284-299

Recent advances in ultrasound diagnosis 5. A. Kurjak, G. Kossoff, eds.

SONOGRAPHIC DEMONSTRATION OF ENDOMETRIAL CHANGES DURING THE MENSTRUAL CYCLE: A CORRELATION WITH SERUM ESTRADIOL AND PROGESTERONE LEVELS

ASIM KURJAK and DAVOR JURKOVIĆ
Ultrasonic Institute, University of Zagreb, "Dr Josip Kajfeš" Hospital, Zagreb, Yugoslavia

INTRODUCTION

In the past several years sonography has become an invaluable research tool for the investigation of spontaneous and induced ovulation and has added to the understanding of folliculogenesis and reproductive endocrinology. Prior to the advent of ultrasound only presumptive evidence of follicular development and ovulation was readily available. Within the context of female endocrinology the uterine cycle is of utmost importance. The major onus of cyclic transformation is borne by the endometrium.

Sonographic assessment of endometrial changes during the menstrual cycle would probably complement and improve ultrasonic evaluation of the ovarian function.

The efficiency of this new promising technique has been demonatrated in several recent reports (4,11,12,13). Furthermore, an excelent correlation of the sonographic measurement of endometrial thickness and histology has recently been described (7).

The aim of the present study was to define the sonographic characteristics of endometrium appearance in the various phases of the menstrual cycle and to correlate them with estradiol and progesterone serum levels.

The clinical significance of the ultrasonically detected endometrial changes in normal and abnormal cycles was also investigated.

SUBJECTS AND METHODS

Endometrial studies were performed in 131 patients who attended infertility clinics for various reasons. Group I included 51 spontaneously cycling women. All cycles in this group were confirmed to be ovulatory in terms of ultrasound and hormonal changes. Group II served as a control group and included 80 spontaneously cycling women who were referred to ultrasound monitoring of follicular growth and detection of ovulation because of suspected abnormality of the menstrual cycle.

In the first group daily ultrasound monitoring of endometrial changes and follicular growth was performed in every patient from day 8-1o (depending on cycle length) until ovulation. A 3.5 MHz real-time sector scanner (Aloka SSD-28o) was used for the purpose. The endometrium was demonstrated in longitudinal and transverse uterine scans, and the maximum anterioposterior diameter of the uterine cavity was measured (Fig. 1).

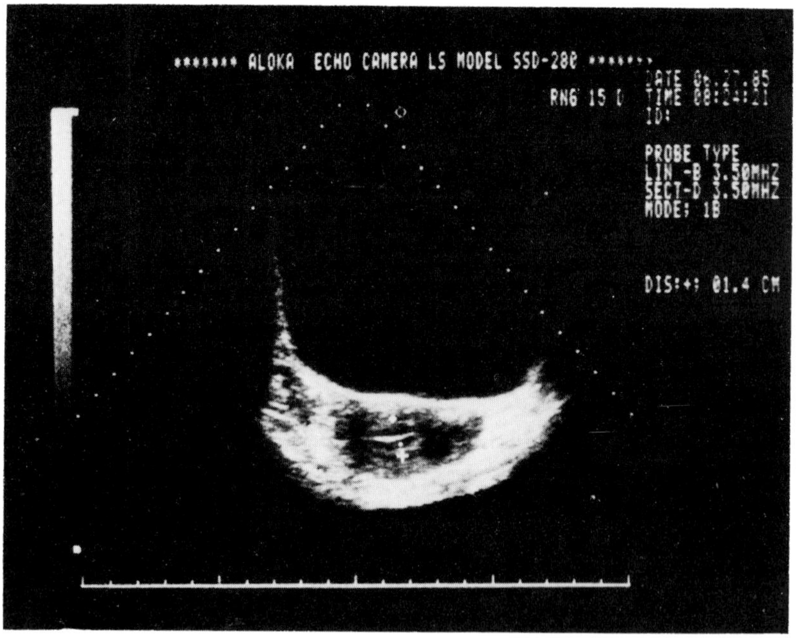

Fig. 1 Transverse sonogram of the uterus illustrating the endometrium in the late proliferative phase and the measurement approach.

The obtained values are obviously twice as high as actual endometrial thickness, but as the measurements are more reliable and accurate, and comparison between various phases of the cycle easier, it was preferred to the measurement of actual endometrial thickness. Changes in endometrium appearance and texture were recognized, and rough sketches drawn daily.

The growing follicles were measured in two planes, and the mean diameter was calculated (Fig. 2). Generally accepted ultrasonic criteria for ovulation were followed (14).

Blood samples were obtained daily prior to ultrasound examinations, and estradiol and progesterone levels were estimated by

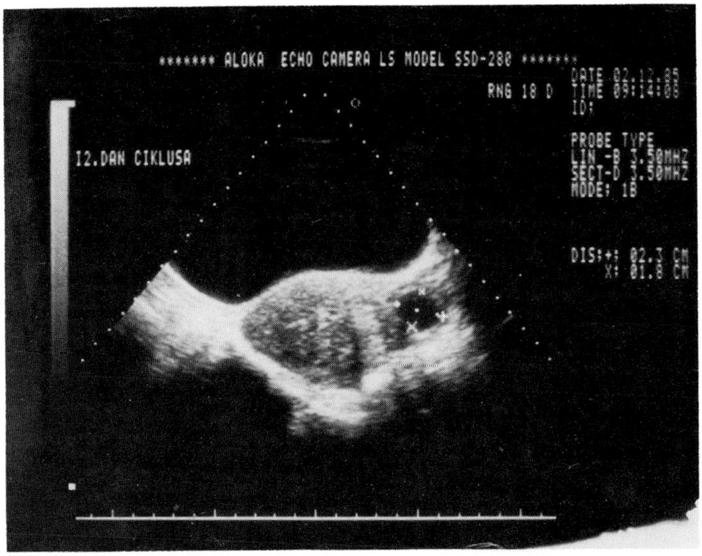

Fig. 2 Sonogram of the left ovary demonstrating a mature ovarian follicle and the measurement technique.

standard radioimmunoassay technique. Following ovulation the patients were examined on days +2, +4, +6 and +8. Endometrial thickness was measured as described above. Blood samples were obtained for progesterone estimations.

Patients in the second group were examined by ultrasound from day 8-1o to ovulation. Endometrial changes and follicular growth were assessed as previously described.

RESULTS

The mean values of all investigated parameters from day -5 to day 0 are shown in Table 1. A clear-cut correlation between serum estradiol and dominant follicle diameter was found (r=o.983; $p < o.ol$) (Fig 3). The correlation between serum estradiol and thickness of the endometrium showed a statistically significant result (r=o.53; $p < o.ol$) (Fig. 4).

In terms of the morphological characteristics of the endometrium in the proliferative and secretory phases, we have defined four distinct types of endometrial appearance. The thin homogeneous

TABLE 1

DAY	ESTRADIOL (pmol/l)	PROGESTERON (nmol/l)	FOLLICULAR DIAMETER (mm)	ENDOMETRIAL THICKNESS (mm)
-5	515,1± 106,8	4,9± 1,81	12,1± 1,3	5,6 ± 2,3
-4	595,1± 140,6	6,9± 2,03	14,1 ± 1,6	7,1 ± 2,1
-3	732,7± 172,2	5,7 ± 1,74	15,3 ± 1,4	8,2 ± 2,5
-2	774,6 ± 241,6	7,3 ± 2,70	17,0 ± 2,1	8,9 ± 1,9
-1	985,3±397,6	8,3 ± 2,21	19,1 ± 2,9	9,8 ± 2,1

Mean values ± SD for all investigated parameters from day -5 to day 0

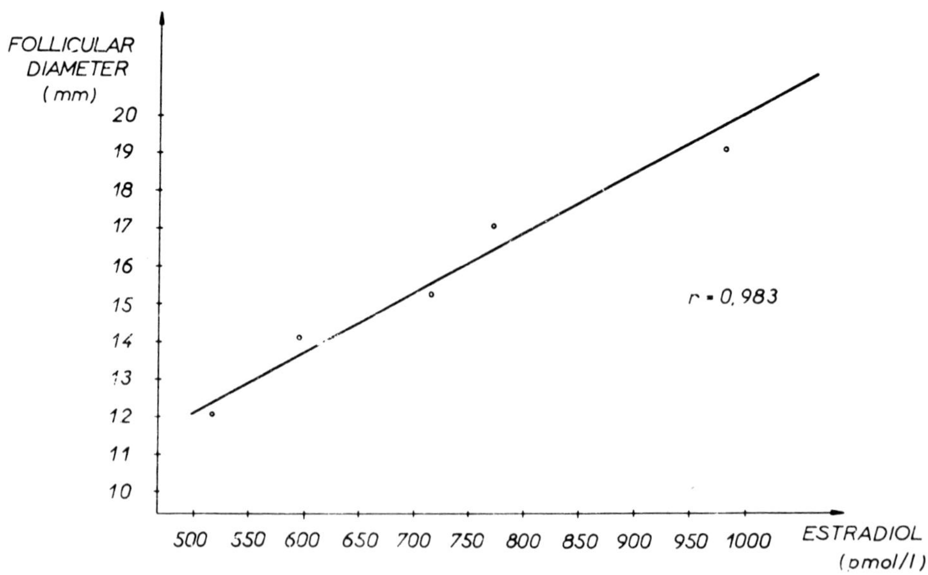

Fig. 3 Diagram showing the correlation of the mean follicular diameter and mean serum estradiol (r= 0.983; $p < o.o1$).

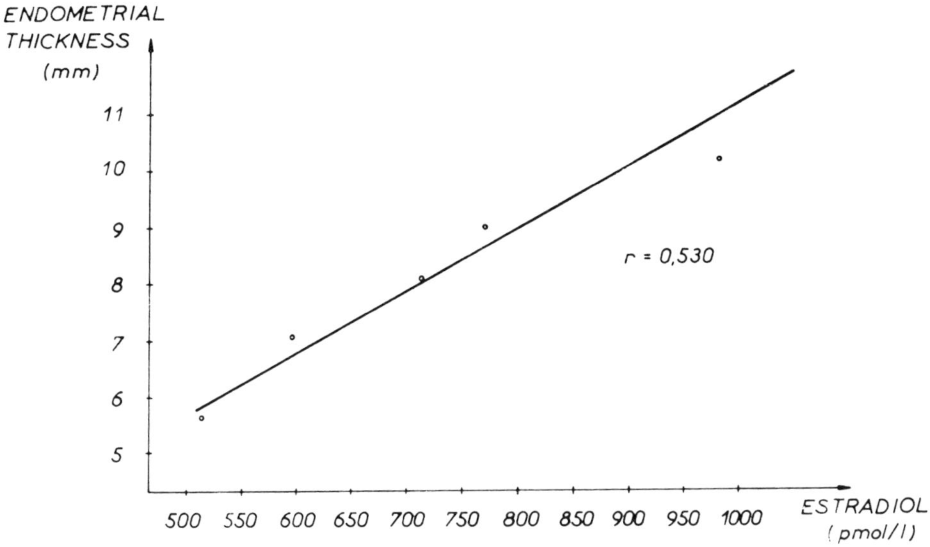

Fig. 4 Diagram showing the correlation of endometrial thickness and serum estradiol in the proliferative phase (r = o.53; p< o.ol)

and echogenic endometrium which can be recognized regularly in early proliferation was designated as Grade 0 (Fig. 5).

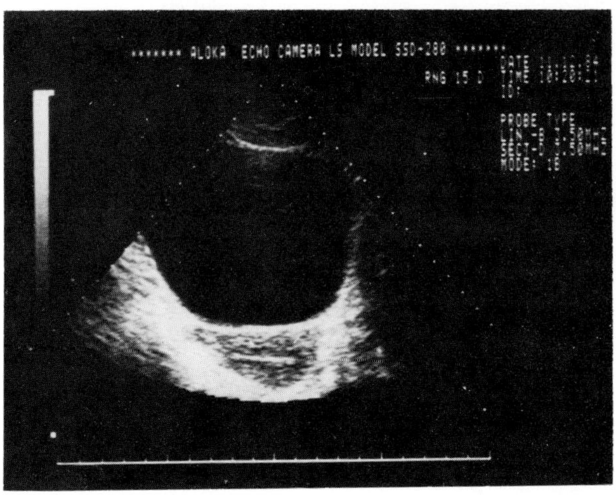

Fig. 5 Transverse sonogram of the uterus in the early proliferative phase illustrating the strong linear echo of the thin and homogeneous endometrium (Grade 0).

The second endometrium type was named Grade I and it is characterized by a thin and well-defined boundary with the myometrium and a marked linear middle echo representing the attached superficial layers of the endometrium (Fig. 6). The endometrium is hypoechoic as compared to the echogenicity of the myometrium. A Grade II endometrium can be distinguished from the previous type by increased echogenicity of the basal portions of the endometrium. The middle echo is less pronounced, but still present (Fig. 7). A Grade III endometrium is generally more echogenic as compared to the myometrium. The middle echo is hardly recognizable or not visible. Grade III appears to be more homogeneous than Grades I and II, and irregularities of configuration can sometimes be recognized (Fig. 8). The grades are shown schematically along with the corresponding values of the other investigated parameters in Table 2.

Statistical analysis showed a significant difference between the established estradiol levels of Grades 0 and I ($t = 3.05$; $p < 0.01$). A significant progesterone level differences were found when Grade I

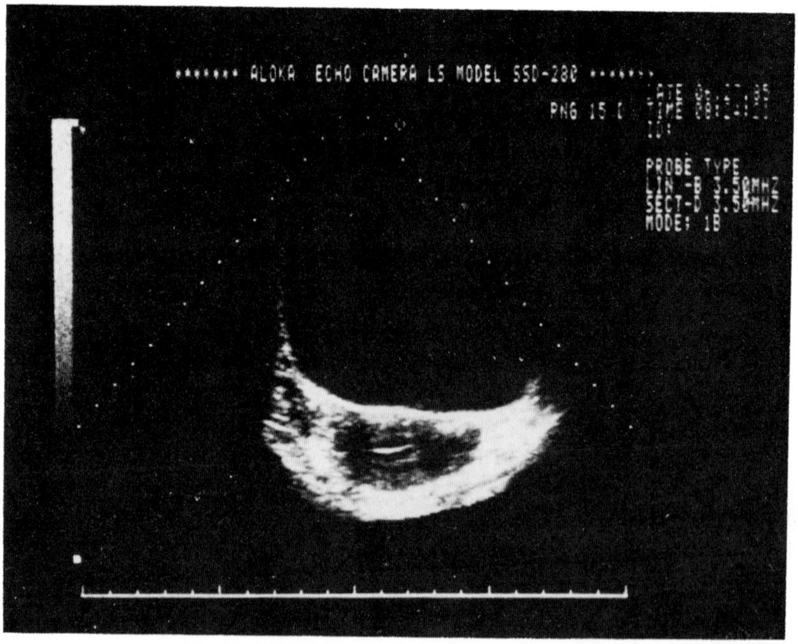

Fig. 6 Moderately thick endometrium with a pronounced linear echo and well defined boundary with the myometrium (Grade I)

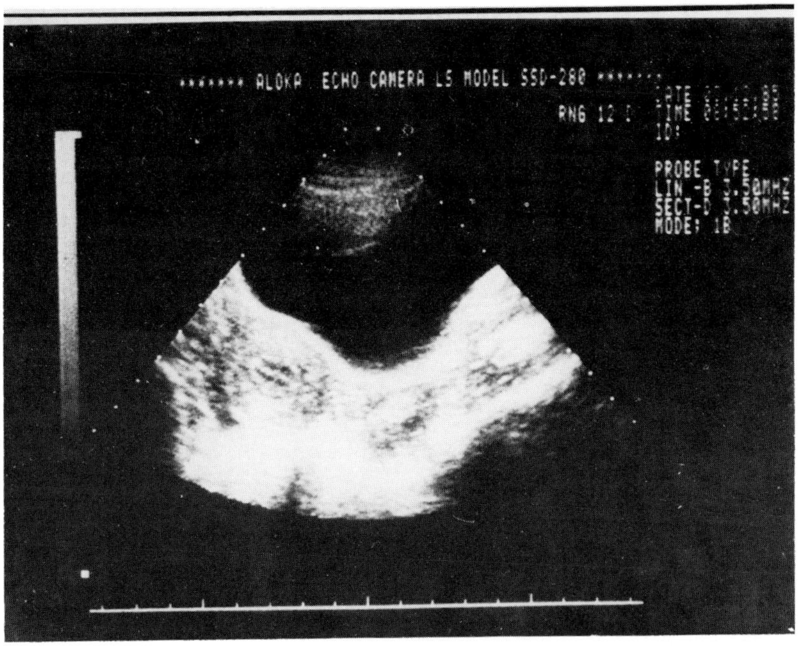

Fig. 7 Increased echogenicity of the basal portions of the endometrium with a preserved linear echo representing the characteristic ultrasonic appearance of the preovulatory endometrium (Grade II).

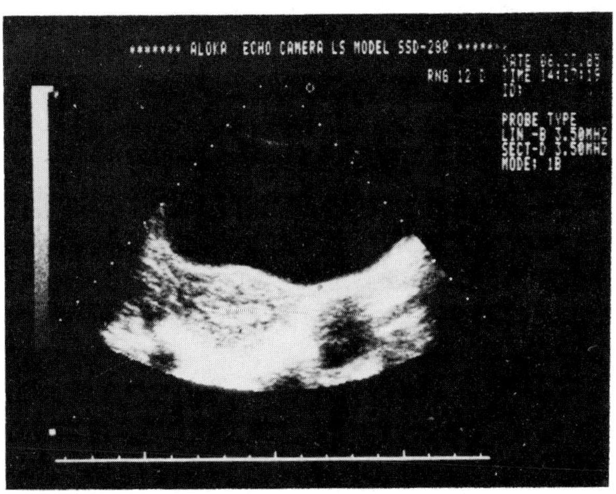

Fig. 8 A thick, echogenic and homogeneous endometrium typical of the secretory phase of the cycle (Grade III).

TABLE 2

GRADE	SKETCH	THICKNESS (mm)	FOLLICULAR DIAMETER (mm)	ESTRADIOL (pmol/l)	PROGESTERONE (nmol/l)
0		1,75 ± 0,70 (1 - 3)	> 10	331,5 ± 117,5	4,7 ± 1,4
I		6,83 ± 2,39 (4 - 12)	16,2 ± 3,4	648,3 ± 306,5	5,1 ± 1,9
II		8,46 ± 1,65 (7 - 14)	18,3 ± 1,9	994,4 ± 345,9	9,4 ± 2,2
III		9,84 ± 3,14 (7 - 16)	19,6 ± 1,4	864,2 ± 324,7	46,3 ± 19,5

Schematic representation of endometrial grades and corresponding values of other investigated parameters (mean ± SD)

and Grade II ($t = 2.72$; $p < 0.01$), and Grade II and Grade III ($t = 5.96$; $p < 0.01$) were compared.

The distribution of the proportion of endometrial grades on days -5, -4, -3, -2, -1 and 0 is shown in Fig. 9. The substantial change in endometrial appearance reflecting the maturity of the preovulatory follicle can be recognized.

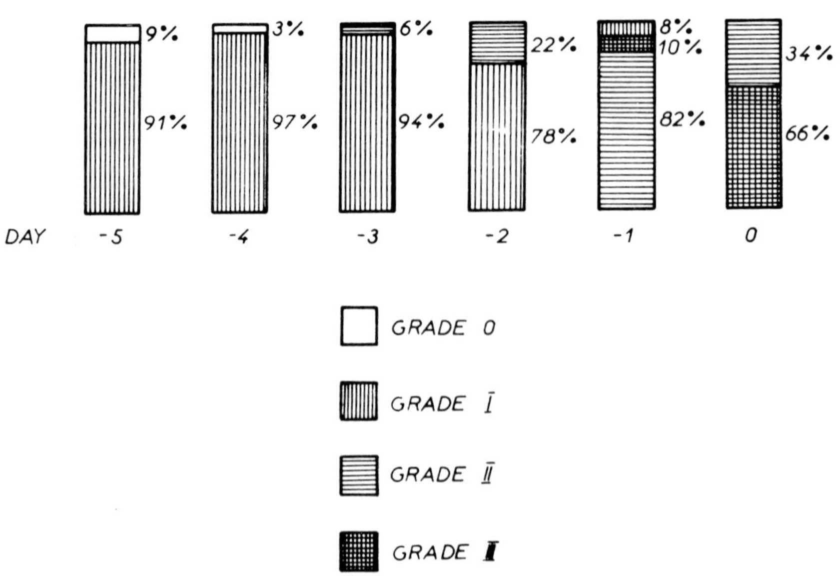

Fig. 9 Distribution of the proportion of visualized endometrial grades from day -5 to day 0.

The results were used to develop a scoring system including both follicular and endometrial assessments in the evaluation of the menstrual cycle (Fig. 1o).

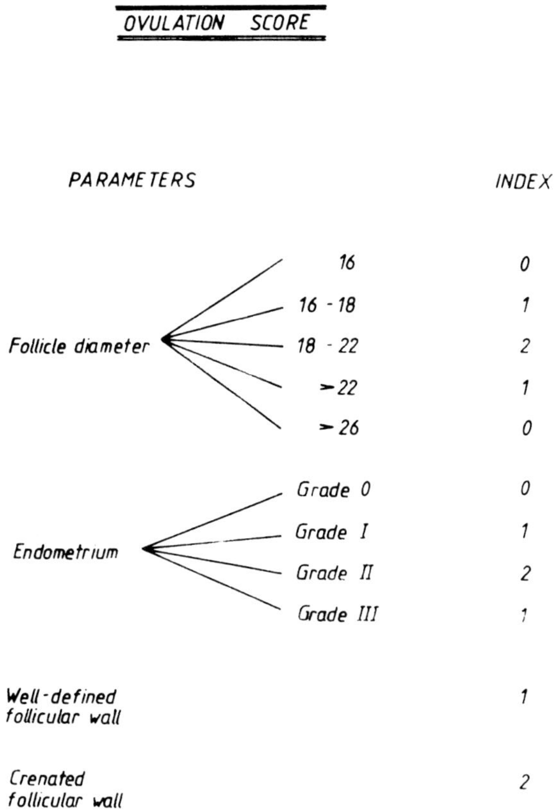

Fig. 1o The scoring system for the evaluation of follicular maturity.

The score was evaluated in the control group. Figure 11 illustrates the daily changes in the ovulation score from day -5 to day -1 in the ovulatory and unovulatory cycles. Test results are shown in Table 3. The score reached values 5-6 in 82% of cases, a day prior to ovulation.

In the secretory phase plasma progesterone and thickness of the endometrium were correlated, but no significant correlation between these two parameters was found ($r = 0.11$; $p > 0.05$).

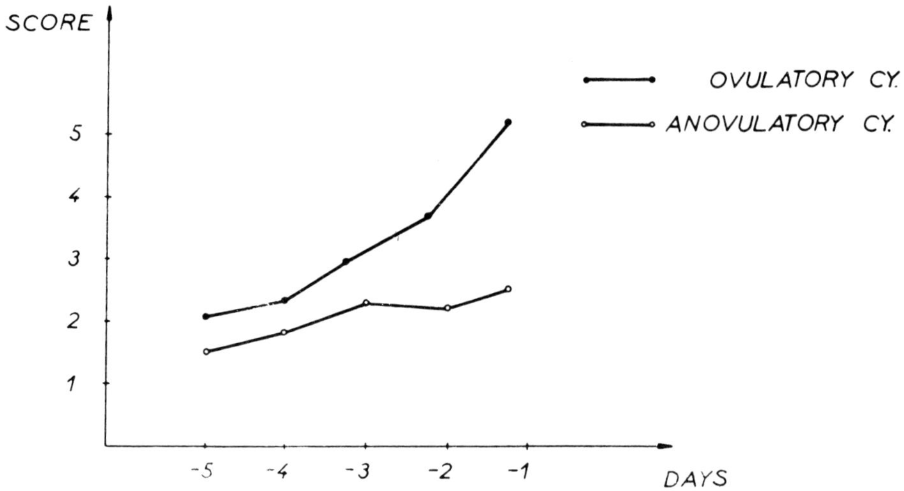

Fig. 11 Diagram showing the daily changes of the score in the ovulatory and unovulatory cycles in the control group.

TABLE III

TEST RESULTS

	SCORE < 5-6	SCORE 5-6
ANOVULATORY CY	32	4
OVULATORY CY	5	36

SENSITIVITY	89 %
SPECITIFICITY	88 %
ACCURACY	88 %

Table 3 Test results of the scoring system in the control group.

DISCUSSION

The endometrium was visualized in 95% of cases in our series. Sonographic visualization proved to be more difficult in retroflected uterus cases and in extremely adipose patients.

The meticulous study of the sonographic appearance of the endometrium showed four main types of endometrial appearance during the menstrual cycle. The comparison of qualitative endometrial appearance changes, with other parameters implies that each grade represents very accurately the relation between estradiol and progesterone production (Table 3). Grade 0 is always associated with low estradiol and progesterone levels and is seen in the early proliferative phase or in cases of serious estrogene deficiency. During the late proliferative phase the linear growth of endometrial thickness which significantly follows the rise in estradiol level has been observed. Grade I endometrium is regularly seen in this phase of the cycle and reflects the pure estrogenic effect on the endometrium. Hackelöer (1984) has reported moderately thick and hypoechoic endometrial appearance in the late proliferation. Low echogenicity of the endometrium was explained by the presence of edematous fluid which separates the stroma cells of the superficial layer (11). The appearance of a Grade II endometrium resembles that of Grade I. The most important feature of this type is increased echogenecity of the basal layer. The endometrium is 7-14 mm thick and the middle echo is less pronounced than in the previous type, but still visible. We strongly believe that this type of endometrium is characteristic for the preovulatory phase of the cycle, and that it reflects the maturity of the ovarian follicle, and the initial rise of progesterone values.

The work of Yussman & Taymor (197o) confirms that there is a rise in plasma progesterone 16 hours before ovulation, following the rise in plasma LH (17). Luteinised granulosa cells, being capable of progesterone synthesis, actually begin to appear prior to follicular rupture (9), which account for the fact that presence of progesterone in the circulating blood can be demonstrated before ovulation. Testard et al. (1982) have recently investigated the concentration of progesterone in the follicular fluid in spontaneous cycles prior and after the onset of LH surge. They found the concentration of progesterone to be five times as high 5-25 hours after the LH surge (16).

Histochemical and biochemical studies have shown the presence of several main substances in the endometrium, e.g., glycogen, ascorbic acid, alkaline glycerophosphatase, β-glucuronidase, nucleic acids and mucopolysaccharides to be cyclic in nature (1). Glycogen is a characteristic element of the progestational phase and, therefore, indicative of the progesterone. Zander & Ober (1962) have detected its presence in the endometria of castrated women as early as two hours following the injection of progesterone

(18). Recent sonographic studies have demonstrated that glycogen is a strongly echogenic substance contributing primarily to the marked echogenicity of the choroid plexus in second trimester fetuses and of the small bowel in children and adults (3,6). The increased echogenicity of the endometrium one day prior to ovulation was associated in our study with significantly higher progesterone lebels and it can therefore serve as a reliable indicator of an LH surge.

The increased echogenicity of the preovulatory endometrium has been recognized by other authors (1o). It has been described as an ultrasound ring-sign appearing as an early gestational sac with an echo free area in the middle. The ring-sign has been demonstrated only in the ovulatory cycles, and the authors suggested its use as an additional parameter that ovulation has taken place.

On the basis of our results we have designed a scoring system which takes into account all ultrasonic parameters for the estimation of follicular maturity. The intrafollicular structure, which has been shown to represent a dissociated cumulus oophorus in the mature follicle, was omitted from the calculation because of the low visualization rate, i.e., less than 15% in our group.

The scoring system was tested in the control group with satisfactory results. Ovulatory cycles can be distinguished from anovulatory cycles with a higher degree of safety as compared to the assessment of follicular growth alone (Fig. 11). By using this system we were able to predict ovulation within next 24 hours with accuracy in 82% of cases. Previous reports, based only on the assessment of ovarian changes, has indicated less reliable results (2).

Endometrial assessment was particularly useful in cases with difficulties in the ultrasonic examination of the ovaries, and in the presence of intraovarian cysts which are sometimes hardly distinguishable from growing follicles, or can alter its shape.

Study of endometrial changes was found to be essential in the diagnosis of certain types of morphological disturbances, in cases of normogonadotropic ovarian insufficiency described by Geisthovel et al. in 1984 (8). The recognition of the progesterone effect on the endometrium associated with the smaller diameter of the growing follicle and irregularities in its shape, was a finding pathognomonic of follicular atresia with luteinization. In our series we have identified 9 patients with this disturbance.

In 4 cases the luteinized unruptured follicle syndrome was diagnosed. In these cases the follicles followed a normal growth pattern and reached a normal preovulatory diameter, but ovulation did not take place and the endometrium showed signs of the progesterone effect. The score showed a decrease after maximum values had been reached in all cases.

In the secretory phase the endometrium is thick and homogeneous (5,7). The endometrial surfaces do not adhere to each other as in the proliferative phase, and the linear echo is therefore lost (15). The endometrium is highly echogenic and clearly visible.

During the secretory phase there was no significant correlation between progesterone levels and endometrial thickness in the group of the ovulatory cycles. The same result can be explained by the marked variability of the progesterone values and a minimal increase in endometrial thickness.

The results of our study indicate the importance of endometrial changes assessment for sonographic evaluation of the ovarian function. It enables better prediction of the ovulation and gives additional data about the functional capability of the growing follicle. Endometrial assessment should be performed regularly, simultaneously with the montoring of the follicular growth, especially in cases of suspected ovarian insufficiency or infertility of unknown reason.

REFERENCES

1. Botella-Llusia J (1973) Endocrinology of woman. In: Saunders WB. Philadelphia, p 265
2. Buttery B, Trounson A, McMaster R, Wood C (1983) Evaluation of diagnostic ultrasound as a parameter of follicular development in an in vitro fertilization program. Fertil Steril 39:458
3. Crade M, Patel J, McQuown D (1981) Sonographic imaging of the glycogen stage of fetal choroid plexus. AJR 137:489
4. Duffield S, Picker R (1981) Ultrasonic evaluation of the uterus in the normal menstrual cycle. Med Ultra 5:7o
5. Feichtinger W (1984) The role of ultrasound in extracorporal fertilization and embryotransfer. In: Kurjak A, Kossoff G (eds) Recent Advances in Ultrasound Diagnosis. Excerpta Medica, Amsterdam, p 224
6. Fleischer AC, Muhletaler C, James AE (198o) Sonographic patterns in normal and abnormal bowel. RCNA 18:145
7. Fleischer AC, Kalemeris GC, Entman SS (1985) Sonographic depiction of the endometrium during normal cycles. In: Gill RW, Dadd MJ (eds) Proceedings of the Fourth Meeting for Ultrasound

in Medicine and Biology. Pergamon Press, Sydney, p 281

8. Geisthövel F, Klosa W, Rabold B, Schillinger H, Breckwoldt M (1984) Further sonographical and endocrine aspects of physiological and insufficient ovarian function. In: Kurjak A, Kossoff G (eds) Recent Advances in Ultrasound Diagnosis. Amsterdam, pp 245-259

9. Guraya SS (1971) Morphology, histochemistry and biochemistry of human ovarian compartments and teroid hormone synthesis. Physiological Reviews 51:785-8o7

1o. Hackelöer BJ (1981) Analysis of five years experience in follicular demonstration. In: Christie AD (ed) Ultrasound and Infertility. Chartwell-Bratt, Bromley, pp 125-145

11. Hackelöer BJ (1984) The role of ultrasound in female infertility management. Ultrasound in Med Biol 1o:35-5o

12. Kurjak A, Jurković D (1985) Demonstration of the uterine endometrial changes during the menstrual cycle. In: Gill RW, Dadd MJ (eds) Proceedings of the Fourth Meeting for Ultrasound in Medicine and Biology. Pergamon Press, Sydney, p 224

13. Nakano H, Sakamoto C, Koyangi T (1982) Endometrial images by ultrasound. Acta Obstet Gynaecol Jpn 34:2

14. Ritchie WGM (1985) Ultrasound in the evaluation of normal and induced ovulation. Fertil Steril 43:167-179

15. Sakamoto C, Nakano H (1982) The echogenic endometrium and alterations during the menstrual cycle. Int J Ginecol Obstet 2o:255

16. Testard J, Castanier M, Feinstein MC, Frydman R (1982) Pituitary and steroid hormones in the preovulatory human follicle during spontaneous or stimulated cycle. In: Rolland R, van Hall EV, Hiller SG, McNatty KP, Schoemaker J (eds) Proceedings of the 4th Reiner de Graaf Symposium. Excerpta Medica, Amsterdam, pp 193-2o1

17. Yussman MA, Taymor ML (197o) Serum levels of follicle stimulating hormone and luteinising hormone and of plasma progesterone related to ovulation by corpus luteum biopsy. J Clin Endocrinol Metabol 3o:396

18. Zander J, Ober GK (1962) Presence of glycogen in the endometria of castrated women following administration of progesterone. Arch Gynäk 196:481

Recent advances in ultrasound diagnosis 5. A. Kurjak, G. Kossoff, eds.

THE QUANTIFICATION OF ULTRASONIC B-MODE IMAGES WITH THE TRIALS OF TISSUE CHARACTERIZATION IN OBSTETRICS AND GYNECOLOGY

MAEDA,K., SAKAO,A., MIO,Y., KIKUKAWA,A., AKAIWA,A. and KIHAILE,P.E.

Department of Obstetrics and Gynecology, Tottori University School of Medicine, Yonago 683 Japan

INTRODUCTION

Although the recent progress of ultrasonic B-mode imaging has been marvellous, and many obstetric and gynecologic diagnoses have been made to clarify several physiological and pathological phenomena which were almost impossible without the ultrasonic method, the diagnoses have been obtained mainly by the analyses of the morphological changes and the biometry data in human body or in the fetus. Since various pre- and post-processings are done in the production of the most clear and useful B-mode image, and also several adjustments are performed in the gain control, STC, FTC, contrast change, etc., many artefacts may devolop in the brightness of B-mode picture of the modern advanced ultrasonic method. In other words, incorrect diagnosis may be possible if the device is controled or adjusted wrongly and the picture is compromised with the artefacts. This is the effect of the semiqualitative control of ultrasonic B-mode machine. Further, the effect will make the beginner complicated in the analysis of the ultrasonograms.

The technique of ultrasonic tissue characterization has been investigated by many researchers in order to aquire more informaions and quantified data in the reflected ultrasound from the living tissue. According to Wells (1977), amplitude analysis which included amplitude measurement, its automatic method, tissue orientation and fluctuation measurement, frequency analysis with the backscattering measurements and backscattering spectra, signal averaging, impediography, correlation technique had been investigated in ultrasonic tissue characterization. Recently, frequency dependent parameter changes, alteration in sound velocity, ultrasonic attenuation in the tissue, etc. are further investigated in ultrasound tissue characterization. Our investigations on the quantification of the reflected ultrasound started in the measurement of reflected ultrasound intensity in radio-frequency (RF) signals, then the intensity histograms of echo brightness level which were obtained with use of an ultrasonographic device, and also by the application of a computer system. Frequency analysis of backscatter and the attenuation measurement are tried preliminarily in the computer analyses in our department. The target of these trials of tissue characterization is the quantification of ultrasonic B-mode image in obstetrics and gynecology.

MANUAL ANALYSIS ON REFLECTED ULTRASOUND AMPLITUDE OF UTERINE MUSCLE AND FIBRO-MYOMATOUS TISSUE

Materials and Methods

The 2MHz ultrasonic generator of the San-Ei UC-10B-1 manual scan B-mode device was modified and used in this study. Electric signal produced at the ultrasound probe terminal was directly connected to the input of Hitachi 15MHz oscilloscope, and the signals were recorded on Polaroid film. RF vibrations were visualized by the technique, then the amplitude of RF wave was measured manually on the film.

The specimens of normal uterine muscle and the fibromyomatous tissue were obtained after medically indicated hysterectomy, and the tissues were prepared into thin square shaped specimen of which size was about 13 x 8 x 2mm. The ultrasound beam was irradiated in the degassed water which was kept in a plastic container in which bottom the Agar mass was accumulated. The Agar mass had a small hole on its surface where the specimen was placed. The long axis of the specimen was adjusted to the ultrasound beam using microadjusting table. The ultrasonic probe diameter was 12.5cm. The distance was 15cm between the ultrasonic crystal and the upper surface of the specimen (Fig. 1).

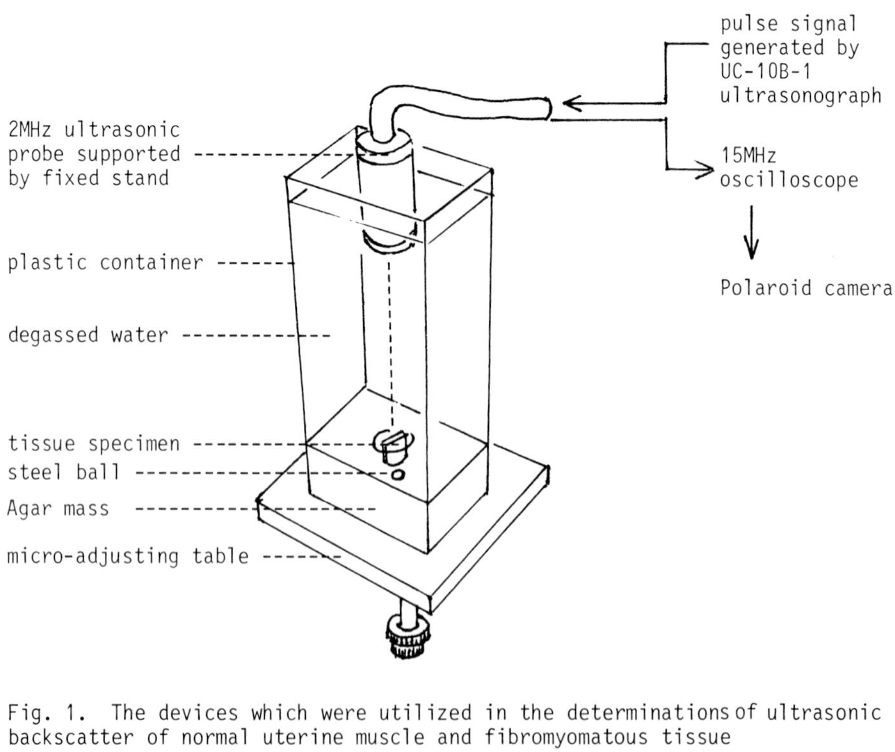

Fig. 1. The devices which were utilized in the determinations of ultrasonic backscatter of normal uterine muscle and fibromyomatous tissue

Results

The amplitude of reflected RF ultrasound was expressed by the value of absolute reflectivity (Rp) which was reported by Ide (1976). A steel ball with the diameter of 3mm was imbeded in the Agar mass, and the amplitude of reflected RF ultrasound from the ball was 13mV on the oscilloscopic screen. Rp of the steel ball was -40dB, since the Rp=log a/x(dB), where "a" is the radius of the ball, and "x" is the distance between the ball and ultrasonic crystal. Rp of specimen was obtained by the comparison of RF voltage to that of the steel ball. The Rp is 20·log 1.3/13 -40(dB), for example, when the RF amplitude of specimen was 1.3mV.

The Rp vlaue of normal uterine muscle tissue was -65.82±6.95 dB in 7 samples, and the range was -72.53 to -65.42 dB, while the Rp of uterine fibromyomatous tissue was -64.13±9.11 dB in 6 smaples in which the range was -68.59 to -58.24dB. Hence, Rp value was significantly larger in uterine fibromyomatous tissue than normal uterine muscle.

The results mean that the reflected RF ultrasound intensity was larger in the myomatous tissue than the normal muscle in quantitative analysis. The fact shows coincidence with common clinical experience which indicates higher echogenicity in uterine fibromyoma than normal uterus. The conclusion also shows the possibility of quantitative diagnosis of B-mode image also in other gynecological tumor. For instance, quantitative analysis and the diagnosis may be possible in some of ovarian malignant tumors in the future.

PIXEL BRIGHTNESS ANALYSIS IN THE ECHO-LEVEL INTENSITY HISTOGRAM

The Ultrasound Intensity Histogram Obtained by a B-mode Device

Methods. Among common ultrasonographs, Aloka 258 prepared the function of intensity histogram analysis. The B-mode image was freezed and stored in the digital scan converter in the form of distributed brightness in every pixel, namely, a pixel stored the intensity of echo-level that was the amplitude of A-mode signal obtained after the detection of reflected RF ultrasound signals. Hence, there was still the possibility of interference caused by the processing of B-mode picture. The controllers of the device were, therefore, adjusted at fixed positions in the study on the histogram.

Linear-scan B-mode image was freezed and the region of interest (ROI) was set on the screen before the analysis of histogram which was then processed in the device, and the result was indicated on the screen at the same time with B-mode picture. X-axis of the histogram showed the 64 grey scales, and Y-axis the normalized percentages of the pixel numbers in every grey scale. Therefore, the histogram shifted to the right when the echo-levels were high, namely, the brightness was high in the ROI. The width of histogram was broad if the ROI included several grades of echo-levels, namely, the image was heterogeneous in the echo-level, and included several levels of A-mode signal amplitude in one ROI.

Materials and Results. In vivo uterine fibromyoma and some ovarian cysts were studied with the A-mode signal intensity histogram. The histogram peak was deviated slightly to the right in the examianton of fibromyomatous tissue if it was compared to normal uterine muscle. The width of the histogram was also broad in uterine fibromyoma. The results were well expected from the investigation of Rp values of RF signals which was reported in previous chapter (Fig. 2).

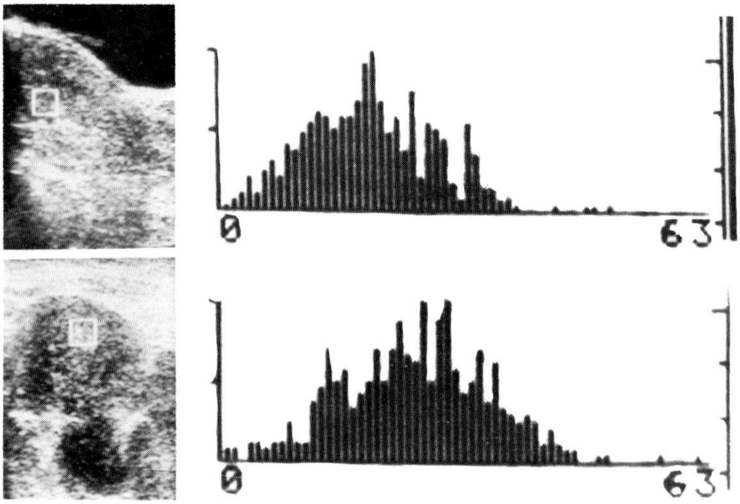

Fig. 2. The comparison of the A-mode signal intensity histograms obtained by Aloka 258 sonograph in normal uterine muscle (upper) and the fibromyomatous tissue (lower). The histograms were shown in negative image to the positive one in the original picture, though the left sided B-mode shows the original ones. Lower Histogram of fibromyomatous tissue shows the peak deviation to the right, and a broad width in the comparison to normal uterine muscle.

A common ovarian cystadenoma and an ovarian dermoid cyst were also compared in the study on the intensity histogram. Usually, these two cysts are well differentiated in the low echogenecity of common cyst and increased brightness in other dermoid cyst. However, the two cystic masses are hardly separated in the B-mode images shown in Fig. 3, because the brightness control was deliberately high in the common cyst image in order to produce the effect of artefact. In spite of such abnormal condition, the histograms show clear difference between these two tissues, namely, intense shift to the right and the broad width of the histogram were noted in the dermoid cyst (Fig. 3). From these results, further study on quantitative analysis was intended in subsequent computer assisted investigation.

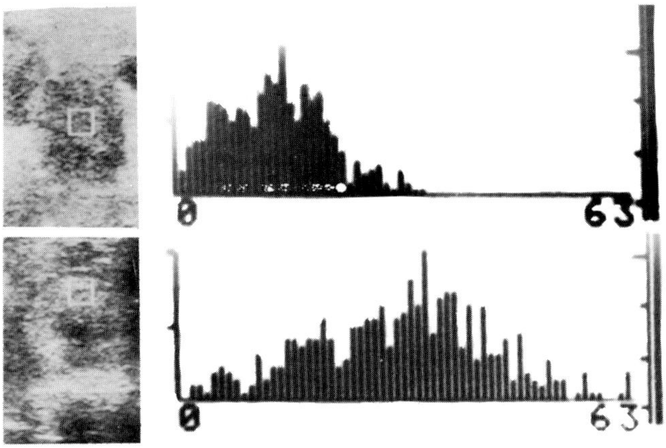

Fig. 3. Upper histogram was obtained in a common ovarian cyst of which B-mode is indicated in the left of the histogram. The B-mode screen was deliberately adjusted to increase the brightness. The lower histogram was obtained in a case of ovarian dermoid cyst, and it shows the shift of its peak to the right and the broader width than the common cyst. The two tissues are well differentiated with the histograms in spite of the artefacts produced in the B-mode image of common ovarian cyst.

The Ultrasound Histogram Assisted by Computer System

Methods. The ultrasonic computer system of our university hospital is Aloka UIP-100, and the system is connected to SSD-270 ultrasonograph. The functions of the computer system are the usual biometries including the length, circumference and area, the volume estimation with repeated area determination in preset interval and their summation, diagnosis of gestational age from the sizes of GS, CRL and BPD, pixel echo-level histogram in multiple ROI with variable circle, quantitative analysis of the histogram, RF signal processings including amplitude determination, power specturm analaysis with the fast Fourier transform (FFT), and the measurement of attenuation.

The function of the anlysis of ultrasonic echo-level histogram is selected in the menu of the software which is displayed on the computer screen. B-mode image is shown in sonographic display, and a ROI is set on the screen under the control of the computer. The histogram is indicated on the B-mode screen simultaneously with quantitative data of the histogram.

Materials and Results. Normal uterine muscle was compared to the uterine fibromyoma in visual analysis of the histogram. The difference was observed in the width of these two histograms (Fig. 4).

The second trial was the analysis of in-vitro B-mode images of expelled placenta which was supported in degassed water, and visualized by B-mode with a linear array transducer placed at the water surface. Placental B-mode images were classified into 3 grades according to the changes. Grade 1 was the most homogeneous, and obtained in relatively early pregnancy, and grade 3 was the most echogenic, heterogeneous and multifoliated. Grade 2 was intermediate between the grades 1 and 3 (Fig. 5).

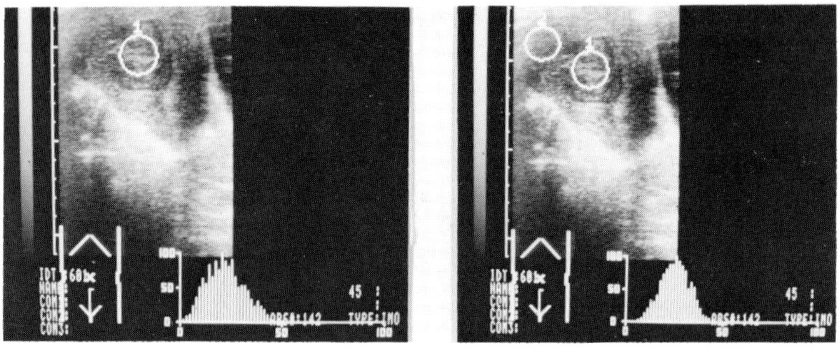

Fig. 4. The histograms were obtained in a case of uterine fibromyoma utilizing SSD-270 sonograph and UIP-100 computer system. The left figure shows the sonogram and echo-level intensity histogram of the fibromyoma node at ROI 1, and the right those of normal uterine muscle at ROI 2. The grey scale of X-axis is normalized into 100 steps. Histogram width is broader in the fibromyoma tissue than the normal muscle.

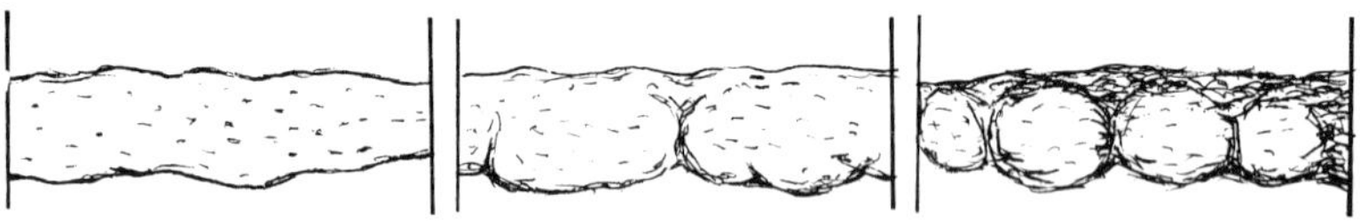

Fig. 5. In-vitro placental ultrasonograms were classified into 3 grades in the present study.

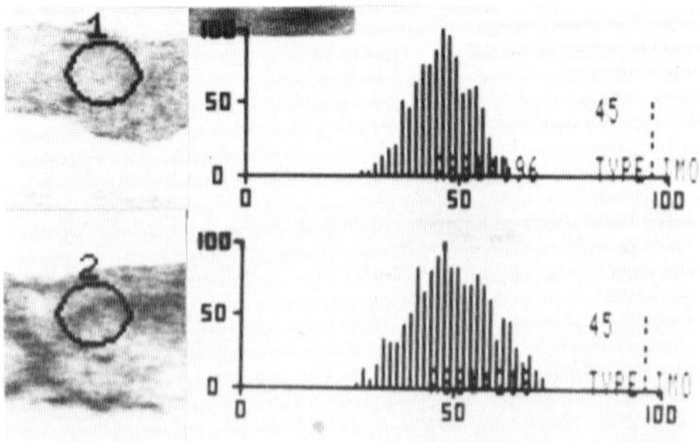

Fig. 6. Computerized echo-level histograms of the placenta in vitro. Upper one was analyzed in the most homogeneous placenta, and the B-mode figure is shown in the left picture. lower one was obtained from the most heterogeneous placenta as shown in the left B-mode image. All figures are shown in negatives.

Every histograms of the echo-levels were normalized in the X-axis expressing the grey scale in 100 steps. Y-axis was also divided into 100, and normalized. The parameters of the histogram in the computerized study including normalized mean grey scale, its deviation and the histogram width were compared at the ROIs which were set at the most heterogeneous parts of the placenta studied in vitro in the grades of 1, 2 and 3 of our classification. The values showed significant difference among the 3 grades of the B-mode picture (Table 1).

Table 1. The difference of the parameters of echo-level histograms obtained in the most heterogeneous parts of B-mode of the placenta in vitro after delivery.

Parameters	B-mode grade		
	1	2	3
Echo-level intensity			
Average	27.69	29.00	39.57
Deviation	18.20	30.20	34.05
Histogram width (%)	40.58	49.95	51.00
N	12	21	17

From these results, structural characteristics was clear among the 3 grades of the placenta studied in vitro. The characterization in the tissue level will be further studied in the future in subsequent statistical investigation and also in the intensity histogram of RF signal of backscattered ultrasound.

The third histographic studies were done on the ovarian follicle and lutein cyst. The follicles before the ovualtion and lutein cysts were compared with the echo-level histograms obtained by the computer analysis. The most homogeneous parts of these two cystic structures showed visual difference in the histograms (Fig. 7).

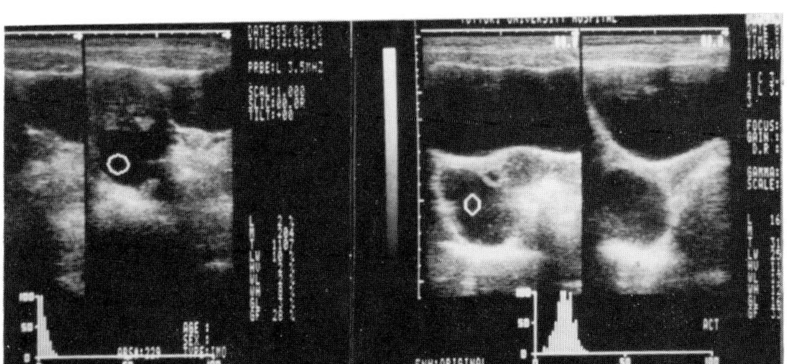

Fig. 7. Computerized echo-level histograms of the contents of ovarian follicle (left B-mode and histogram) and lutein cyst (right ones). There can be seen clear visual difference in the two histograms.

Statistical studies on the histograms of ovarian follicle and lutein cyst showed the difference in the echo-level and histogram width (Table 2). The result shows the utility of the histogram in the studies on preovulatory follicle, post-ovulatory changes and abnormal ovulatory processes.

Table 2. Analytic and statistical studies on the histogram parameters obtained in the contents of preovulatory ovarian follicle and lutein cyst.

Parameters	Follicle (N=10)	Lutein cyst (N=10)
Echo-level average	1.74±0.41	9.06±5.90
deviation	1.04±0.56	13.25±5.05
maximum	5.80±1.60	21.83±4.87
minimum	1.00±0.00	3.16±2.13
Histogram width	9.20±2.38	29.16±5.19

RADIO-FREQUENCY ANALYSIS OF BACKSCATTER ULTRASOUND

The reflected RF ultrasound was also studied with use of the UIP-100 computer system. An in-vitro placenta was used in the preliminary investigations on the RF signal analysis. The trial was successful, and further studies are scheduled on various materials in the fields of obstetrics and gynecology (Fig. 8).

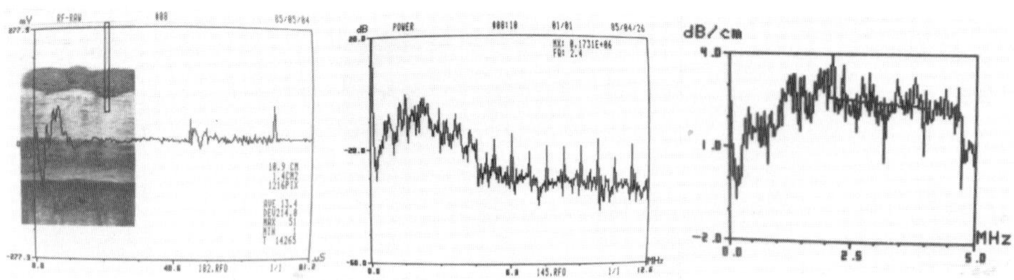

Fig. 8. The RF ultrasound analysis on the backscatter of in-vitro placenta. The narrow area of the placenta was analyzed as shown in the B-mode image.
Left; amplitude of RF signal. Middle; frequency analysis of the backscatter with FFT. Right; ultrasound attenuation is studied by the curve which was obtained by the difference of 2 power spectra.

REFERENCES

1. Ide, M. (1976) Steel ball method for the measurement of overall sensitivity of ultrasonic diagnostic equipment. Jpn J Med Ultrasonics 3:45-52

2. Wells, P.N.T. (1977) Biomedical Ultrasonics. Academic Press, London, New York, San Francisco

INDEX OF AUTHORS